True Calling

Inspirational Stories and Resources for Caregivers

by
Laura Marie Patterson

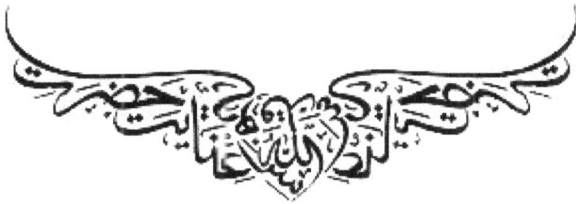

www.TrueCallingBook.com

iBookMusic Publishing
Printed in the U.S.A.

True Calling: Inspirational Stories and Resources for Caregivers
Authored by Laura Marie Patterson and edited by Becky Nelson

ISBN-13: 978-0615425573
ISBN-10: 0615425577

iBookMusic Publishing
1250 Oakmead Pkwy. Suite 210
Sunnyvale, CA. 94089 USA

phone (408) 462-1092
fax   (888) 872-4451
info@ibookmusic.com
www.ibookmusic.com

First Edition
June 2011

The following stories were written from the true experiences of the author. Some of the names and locations may have been changed to protect privacy.

True Calling
Laura Marie Patterson

Table of Contents

Forward: **Introduction**

Section 1 **True Stories of Caregiving Experiences**

Chapter 1: **Change in Career**   8

Chapter 2: **Jimmy and Sabrina - Their Commitment**   14

Chapter 3: **Matthew - Finding Comfort in Food**   22

Chapter 4: **Kathy - A Family in Turmoil**   40

Chapter 5: **William - Building Trust**   70

Chapter 6: **Francis - Finding Closure**   102

Chapter 7: **Sam - His Strong Will to Live**   132

Chapter 8: **Maxine - Coping With Loss**   138

Chapter 9: **Dave - A Family Caregiver's Prospective**   146

Table of Contents

Section ll –   **Family and Caregiver Resources**

Appendix A: **Building Trusting Relationships**   158

Appendix B: **Safety in the Home and Hidden Dangers**   162

Appendix C: **Nutrition and Food Preparation**   166

Appendix D: **Dementia and Memory Loss**   170

Appendix E: **Exercise and Social Activities**   176

Appendix F: **Working With Family Members**   182

Appendix G: **Supporting Loss and Grief**   186

Appendix H: **Caring for the Caregiver**   194

Acknowledgments   198

This Living Book will continue to grow with the shared experiences of it's readers. Please join us online: **www.TrueCallingBook.com** and share your experiences.

This page was left blank intentionally.

Forward - Introduction

*I*f someone would have told me 20 years ago that I would now be writing a book about my caregiving experiences, my reply would have been ..

"You must be mistaking me for somebody else!"

Growing up in Southern California and playing the guitar at an early age, my career ambitions were initially focused on the music industry. As a songwriter, singer and performer, I experienced professional success as a young adult.

The age of home computers in the 1980's sparked a strong interest in programming. First as a hobby, then later as a career choice. I worked for several pioneering companies that were responsible for the early development of the Internet. This was an exciting time in my life filled with travel and financial rewards.

With the dawn of the New Millennium, a series of unforeseen events lead to a new and unexpected career path. What was to be a temporary position soon became a work of passion and rewarding experiences. Each client wrote a new and unique chapter in my life. As I would tell these stories to family and friends, it became apparent that I had finally found my true calling.

I dedicate this book to all the special people that I had the opportunity of sharing a chapter in their lives and in doing so enriched my life forever.

Laura Marie Patterson

Chapter 1

A Change in Career

*M*y application and background checks are now complete as I eagerly await a call from my new agency and my first caregiving assignment. I reflect back on the circumstances that had brought me to this crossroad in my career and the decision that would not only change my life, but also touch the lives of those placed in my care.

caregiving was to be a drastic departure from my previous career as a software engineer. Although challenging, sitting within the confines of the cubicle for many hours a day leaves little time for social interaction.

Living and working in Hawaii was an enjoyable experience. The beautiful beaches and spectacular sunsets were a welcome break from the daily stress and demands required of my job. Unfortunately, with the Internet downturn and the eventual sell off of the company I worked for, I had to leave this island paradise for the mainland in search of new employment opportunities.

After arriving in the San Francisco Bay area and the heart of the Silicon Valley, my worst fears were realized. The dot com crash was indeed nationwide and with no computer jobs available. This reality prompted a visit to the state employment office where I began my job search in earnest for alternative job opportunities in the area.

Change in Career
Laura Marie Patterson

In looking over the various job postings, one in particular caught my attention. It was from an health care agency that offered free training and placement for caregivers. This was of interest to me since I had worked in a hospital during my college years and found the experience very rewarding. After all, this would just be a temporary position until the demand for software engineers improves. I made the call later that afternoon. The call that would change my life forever.

I was told that training classes were to begin the following week. I was to stop by their office and fill out the necessary paperwork in order to secure my seat in the upcoming classes. I drove to their offices in eager anticipation.

Upon my arrival to the agency's small but efficient office, I was asked to fill out an application and other required forms. I was also given an informational packet about the caregiving position. I took this home and later read through its contents.

A description of duties that is required of a caregiver was enclosed. These tasks included bathing, dressing, preparing the clients meals, shopping, laundry, light housekeeping and in some cases transportation to and from the clients appointments.

As I read over the list of assignments, the position seemed to describe that of a caretaker and not what I imagined of a caregiver. Certainly companionship and moral support would be an essential part of caregiving?

Since the class was scheduled to begin the following week, all my questions would then be answered. I looked forward to being active participant in the class and to learn more about the caregiving experience.

True Calling
Laura Marie Patterson

The following Monday was met with eager anticipation as I entered the classroom. The seats were filled mostly with women representing various ages and ethnic groups. I took my seat at the rear of the classroom just as the teacher had arrived. She was an attractive middle aged woman, professionally dressed and carrying an armload of folders.

She introduced herself as Margaret, a Registered Nurse and Healthcare Administrator. She asked each of us to introduce ourselves starting at first row of chairs and then moving around the classroom.

The folders were passed around the room as she explained the topics that the class would cover. These included many of the tasks that were outlined in the information that I received from the agency. We were also told to purchase a workbook that would be the basis of our class curriculum.

Each class discussed a new chapter in the book that we have previously read at home. The proper use of body mechanics for non-ambulatory clients was demonstrated. We also had some guest speakers discussing such topics as nutrition and proper bathing techniques. Upon graduation I was confident in the basic skills of caregiving and ready for my first hands on experience with a client.

My thoughts were now disrupted by the ringing of my telephone. It was Ann from the agency with my first caregiving assignment. I was to work with a couple that lived in a large apartment building just down the street from my home.

Change in Career
Laura Marie Patterson

I was to report at 10:00 am the next morning and was advised that the husband Jimmy had just been released from the hospital where he had a heart bypass procedure. His wife Sabrina suffered from epilepsy since childhood and was also confined to a wheelchair.

Later that night I found it hard to sleep as my mind was filled with nervous anticipation, for tomorrow will be my first day as a caregiver.

This page was left blank intentionally.

Chapter 2
Jimmy and Sabrina - Their Commitment

Chapter 2

Jimmy and Sabrina - Their Commitment

*T*he morning sun played host to a lovely Spring day as I walked the short distance to my first caregiving assignment. Upon reaching the building I noticed a phone at the entrance with listings of the each of the residents and a button to phone them. I looked down the list, found my client's names and pushed their button. After several rings I was greeted by a man's weak voice and a faint hello. I introduced myself as their new caregiver sent by the agency and was promptly buzzed in.

I walked down the long hallway lined with doors looking for their apartment number. I felt my heart beat a little faster as I began to feel nervous for the first time. As I approached their door I saw that it was already cracked open. As I stuck my head inside to say hello, I noticed the TV in the living room was on with two recliners facing away from the door. I said hello loudly as to be heard over the sound of the TV. In return I heard a woman's voice say, "Come on in honey."

As I entered the room both had their attention focused on the television. I introduced myself and repeated that I was to be their new caregiver. The woman then introduced herself, "Hello, I'm Sabrina and this is my husband Jimmy."

Sabrina looked much younger than her husband. Her long dark hair framed her rounded face and was parted to one side slightly hiding one of her large brown eyes. Her skin was pale white and smooth, as she appeared to be in her 30s.

In stark contrast, Jimmy was a thin frail man with gray hair and thick eye glasses. His advanced age and failing health was apparent in his appearance.

Jimmy just stared straight ahead as he continued watching the program as I replied,

"Nice to meet you both."

Sabrina then turned to join her husband without saying another word. I stood there for several minutes before sitting on the couch across from the two and remained there quietly until their program finished.

Jimmy turned off the TV as he turned to me abruptly and said,

"I sent the last three packing "

"Excuse me?", I replied inquisitively.

With a stern look he barked back, "They were all worthless so I sent them home!"

Jimmy stood up from his chair grasping his cane as he made his way into the bedroom slamming the door behind him. Sabrina looked embarrassed as she apologized for Jimmy's behavior.

True Calling
Laura Marie Patterson

"I'm sorry Laura, Jimmy is not comfortable with having anyone else around. Since his return from the hospital he has been very protective of me. You see Laura, it's always been Jimmy that has taken care of me. Please have patience with him. I'm sure you will work out just fine."

"That's okay Sabrina", I replied with a smile. "This is only my first day. We will all get to know each other better in time. Should I check on your husband?"

Sabrina looked over at the bedroom door then back at me as she replied, "it's okay, Jimmy is tired and it's time for him to rest. You can check in on him after awhile but for now, let's just have a talk."

"Can I get you something to drink? Maybe a cup of tea?"

"Sure, thank you", Sabrina replied." The pot is on the stove and the tea bags are in the left side cabinet."

On my way to their small kitchen, I noticed the many photos that hung on the living room walls. Obviously these photos where taken over the many years of their marriage. There were also some family photos of what appeared to be Sabrina with her parents when she was a child.

As I entered the room carrying the tray with our tea, I noticed Jimmy had sat back in his recliner and was now facing in my direction.

"I am sorry Laura for my outburst, I have not been feeling myself lately."

"That's okay Jimmy. It is perfectly understandable with all that you have been through. Can I get you a cup of tea or something to drink?" Jimmy replied with a smile, "No thank you. So, tell us about yourself Laura."

I began to recount the events that brought me to their home. I explained that the two of them were my first caregiving assignment. "Please go easy on me!", I said with a light chuckle. Jimmy with a serious face replied, "Well.. Your still here aren't you?, I guess you have passed the first test!" With that statement we all laughed.

The weeks and months that followed were filled with talks, laughter, activities and outings. We would sometimes take our walks to a nearby park and carry a picnic lunch. Since their apartment was just around the corner from the market, all three of us would often go shopping together. Jimmy would coin our group collectively as "The Curiosity Train", for the funny looks that we would receive as Jimmy would lead us using his walker, Sabrina following close behind him in her motorized wheelchair and myself acting as the "caboose" pushing a cart filled with groceries. Jimmy had suggested on several occasions that he needed to get himself an engineer's cap. Jimmy certainly had an unique since of humor!

One morning on my way to their apartment I noticed several emergency vehicles out in front of their building. Since there were several residents living in the building, I did not immediately connect them to Jimmy and Sabrina. As I entered the building and approached their apartment it became apparent the response team was indeed for one of them. A neighbor was standing just outside their door and yelled out to me, "it's Jimmy." As I made my way into their apartment, I could see Jimmy as he lay on the floor.

True Calling
Laura Marie Patterson

Sabrina was sitting in her chair and appeared to be in a state of shock. She had not even noticed that I had entered the room as I reached for her shoulder. "Sabrina, I am here, what happened?" As if coming out of a trance, she looked up at me with tear filled eyes, "he just fell to the ground so I called 911. Is he going to be okay?"

"Sabrina, Jimmy is in good hands."

On the count of three the attendants lifted Jimmy on to the stretcher. I asked one of them where they were taking him? "Ma'am, we are air lifting him to Stanford Hospital." They carried Jimmy out to the awaiting helicopter that had landed on the roof of their large building. I sat with Sabina on couch with my arms around her she began to sob as she asked, "Laura, what will become of me if something happens to Jimmy?"

"Jimmy is one his way to one of the top hospitals in the country. Meanwhile, I will remain here with you until we get word of his condition then I will make arrangements for you to go see him, okay?"

"Thank you Laura. It's so good to have a friend like you at a time like this."

Sabrina's words reached to the core of my heart as I realized the important role that I was playing in both her and Jimmy's life.

"Sabrina I need to use your phone to make a couple of calls. I need to call my office to make arrangements for your overnight care while Jimmy is away and then I will call the hospital. Are you okay? Can I get you something?"

"I just want my Jimmy!", as she continued to sob.

Later that day we received a call from the hospital. Jimmy has been moved to the cardiac care floor and was in stable condition. He had a minor stroke, a complication of his previous bypass surgery. Sabrina's quick response in calling 911 was a major factor in saving Jimmy's life. We would go to the hospital the next day and several days over the following two weeks until Jimmy was released back home.

Shortly after Jimmy's stroke, the county that was providing their care giving services through my agency, decided that it would be best that Jimmy and Sabrina relocate from their independent living building with a caregiver to a supervised 24 hour care facility. Neither of them were happy about the counties decision however, in the best interest of safety and to better monitor their heath-care needs, it was the best possible recommendation for the both of them.

I think of Jimmy and Sabrina often. Their strong love and commitment for one another was inspiring and the experience I had gained from this assignment was invaluable.

True Calling
Laura Marie Patterson

Chapter 2 Jimmy and Sabrina - Their Commitment

Resource Index

Appendix A: Building Trusting Relationships 158

Appendix F: Working With Family Members 182

Related Chapters

Chapter 5: William - Building Trust 70

Chapter 9: Dave – A Family Caregiver's Perspective 146

Chapter 3
Matthew - Finding Comfort in Food

Chapter 3

Matthew - Finding Comfort in Food

*A*fter working exclusively with Jimmy and Sabrina over the last 10 months, the agency would assign to me up to five different different clients per week. One of those clients was a 40 year old man named Matthew living with his elderly mother in their small home.

Matthew has been plagued with a serious eating disorder for many years. His weight had ballooned to over 500 pounds and was impacting both his physical health and his ability to live independently. His extreme weight gain made it nearly impossible for him to perform normal daily activities and he required a special breathing machine when he slept at night. I was assigned to this case four hours daily, three times a week. I was to provide help with his bathing, exercise and meal preparation.

Upon my arrival at their home, I was greeted by a petite elderly woman that introduced herself as Betty, Matthew's mother.

"Hello, nice to meet you. My name is Laura and I was sent by the agency to assist your son Matthew."

"Come in my dear, Matt is still in bed sleeping. Won't you have a seat in the front room. Can I get you something?"

"No thank you Betty, I am fine. When does your son normally awaken?"

"It depends. He did not sleep very well last night. To be honest with you Laura, I am very worried about my Matt."

The look of concern was written all over her face as she to continued to explain the many attempts to control his weight even to the point of stomach surgery. "He cares more about food than his own health and it is killing him!" As she continued the tears began to roll down her tired eyes. "I just don't know what to do anymore. I love him and he is my son, but he refuses to help himself."

Laura: I can see that your a caring and loving mother, but even the best of intentions require cooperation. Possibility there is something I can do to help? Has he ever been to counseling or a support meeting?

Betty: He has been to several behavioral therapists, but has never opened up to any of them. His weight has been up and down since his adolescence.

Laura: Over eating like other types of addictions are often a symptom of a deeper emotional problem. Just like alcoholics, there are support groups for compulsive over eaters. Has anyone ever suggested he attend one?

Betty: I don't believe he has ever been to one. Possibly you could suggest a meeting to Matt?

Laura: Sure, first I will let Matthew become comfortable with me otherwise, the suggestion may make him feel awkward.

Betty: Thank you Laura. I think I will wake Matt and let him know your here. Let's keep this discussion between us, okay?

True Calling
Laura Marie Patterson

Laura: Of course Betty. I really appreciate your candidness about Matthew and I look forwarded to getting to know him.

Betty excused herself and headed down the hall on her way to her son's room. I thought about Matthew's refusal to confide in the therapist and wondered if he would be willing to confide in me. It will be hard to make a real difference in Matthew's life with the limited time I will have with him each day.

I could hear the distant whispers as Betty was waking Matthew. "Matt, your caregiver is here.. you should get up now." In response I could only hear Matthew's grumbling. After a few minutes Betty returned.

Betty: I'm sorry Laura, Matt will be up shortly. It takes him some time to get himself out of bed.

Laura: Should I help him with anything?

Betty: Matt is somewhat embarrassed. He was expecting a male caregiver.

Laura: I see, should I call my office to see if they can send a male caregiver to assist him?

Betty: No Laura, I think you may be best for Matt. Let's give it a try, okay?

I told Betty I would be happy to help her son in any way possible and then headed to Matthew's room. I knocked on his door..

"Good Morning Matthew, my name is Laura. I am here to give you a hand. I know this may be a bit awkward for you." A deep voice loomed from behind the door, " just a second, I am putting my robe on." The door soon opened and out walked Matthew. A very large man indeed, but with a gentle ease about him.

"Nice to meet you Matthew. Since this is our first day and I don't know your normal routine, do you mind guiding me along?"

"Well.. first I will wash up. Do you mind fixing me something to eat? My mom will show you where everything is at"

"Certainly", I said with a smile. "Just let me know if you need any help."

I could hear Betty already in the kitchen with the pots and pans rattling as I headed down the hallway.

Laura: What does Matthew usually have for his breakfast?

Betty: He likes his frosted corn flakes first, then he will either have 3 eggs with toast or pancakes and bacon.

Laura: That does not sound like a very healthy diet for a man in his condition.

Betty: I know Laura. I have tried to get him to get a smaller and healthier breakfast but if I don't give him what he wants, then he will eat whatever he can find in the cabinets.

True Calling
Laura Marie Patterson

Laura: Like what?

Betty: Like chips, cookies, and even candy.

Laura: Do you mind my asking who has been doing the shopping?

Betty: Well, lately I have been driving to the corner market and picking up a few items during the week. I had a friend's daughter do the shopping on the weekends before she left for college. That is partially why your here Laura. In addition to his personal care, I was hoping you could assist with the shopping as well?

Laura: Of course Betty that is part of my duties. I must say however, it is also my responsibility that Matthew eats a healthy diet. Many of the clients I have worked with have special dietary requirements. Matthew's diet plan should be based around low fat high protein foods and restricted sugar. Does Matthew like fruit?

Betty: He does like bananas and strawberries sprinkled with sugar.

Laura: Bananas sound okay and strawberries are fine, but the sugar is a absolute no-no. Do you have any of these in the house?

Betty: No, we need a lot of food items. Could you possibly do some shopping today for us?

Laura: Sure, but first I would like to discuss a food plan with Matthew and suggest some healthier choices. Let's get his breakfast ready and while he is eating I will make a grocery list.

Betty: Sounds great Laura! I am so glad your here to help out with all of this, as I just do not have the energy anymore.

Laura: I am happy to be here and I will do my best to help start Matthew with his diet.

As Betty and I was preparing Matthew's breakfast, I could hear him enter the living room and turn on the T.V. Betty told me that she brings his breakfast on a tray and he eats in the recliner that also has a built-in lift to assist him in getting up. I brought in the tray with his cereal, one piece of toast and two eggs. I could immediately see the look on Matthew's face as he saw the portions that were provided to him.

Matthew : Where is my bacon? and I always have 3 eggs with my breakfast!

Laura: I am sorry Matthew, you are low on groceries right now. While you are eating I thought we would make a shopping list together and do some meal planning?

Matthew: Fine by me. I need plenty of hamburger meat since I like my burgers for lunch. We just buy the large family pack since it is less expensive than buying the small individual packages.

Laura: An occasional hamburger is fine but I would suggest ground sirloin since it is much lower in fat than ground beef. Also, having variety for your lunch would be better. Would you agree?

Matthew: Laura since it's your first day I will go easy on you, but I do have my limits!

True Calling
Laura Marie Patterson

I could see by the expression on Matthew's face that he was not comfortable with my intervention. This was to be a difficult transition for him and all my efforts in getting him to eat a healthy diet will be in vain if he is not a willing participant. I will make these changes gradually and temper them with positive reinforcement. Baby steps in the right direction will eventually make a difference. If I push to hard he will not accept my help and refuse my services.

Laura: Okay Matthew, I am sorry. Please understand, I work with many different clients and each of them have their own dietary requirements. My only intention is to get to know the kinds of foods you enjoy and to assist you in making healthy choices. Can we meet somewhere in the middle?

Matthew: Many have tried to control my diet in an effort to help me to lose some weight but even loosing 100 pounds would barely make a dent in my 500 plus total weight!

Laura: I can't begin to imagine how hard life must be for you, but doing nothing is not the solution. Even my best intentions will make no difference unless you want change your life style for the better. I am here to support you in your difficult journey but you must be willing to take the steps necessary.

Matthew: So what is your suggestion Laura?

Laura: Let's begin by making some simple substitutions. For example, instead of the sugar frosted flakes, how about plain flakes with bananas or strawberries?

Matthew: No sugar? I don't know about that!

28

Laura: Then we could add a small amount of sweetener such as Splenda. How does that sound?

Matthew: Okay, I will try that.

As we developed a meal plan together, I would flag the high fat and carbohydrate items and suggest a way to replace them with a healthier choices. Soon our shopping list was complete and a 7 day meal plan was developed. After finishing the breakfast dishes I headed to the super market with my shopping list in hand. Knowing that Matthew was a party to the meal plans was a great first step. However, realizing that bad eating habits are difficult to break, this is going to be a difficult challenge.

After returning from the market, I organized the groceries and then joined Matthew in the living room.

Laura: Mission accomplished! We are all set with our menu for the week. I will prepare your breakfast and lunch while your mother will make your dinner for you. Not only do we need to modify your diet but portion control is equally important.

Matthew: So now your going to starve me too?

Laura: Not quite, but we have to limit your calories in order for you to loose weight. Also, exercise is another important component.

Matthew: You mean weight lifting and such?

True Calling
Laura Marie Patterson

Laura: Not quite. I suggest walking for starters. After breakfast a short walk and in the afternoon as well. Not far at first, but slowly build our distance over time. Agreed?

Matthew: Okay, but it is hard for me to walk so we will have to take it slow.

From that very first day in working with Matthew, we both developed a mutual respect. I was determined to show Matthew that we could work towards his elusive goal of losing the weight needed to regain control of his life. Although we only had four hours daily together, we worked out a schedule which included his walks. He slowly adapted to a healthier diet with smaller portions. Betty was pleased with her son's progress with guarded enthusiasm for the disappointment she had experienced in the past. We did not have a scale at his home in which to weigh him, so we had to wait until his monthly doctor appointment.

The first month Matthew lost approximately 25 pounds which was less than we both anticipated however, "every pound lost is a still a victory", as I would later explain to him. I also noticed a change in Matthew's attitude and personality. He did not seem as cheerful and talkative as when we first met. After breakfast one morning I talked to him about what I had observed.

Laura: Do you mind if I ask you something Matthew?

Matthew: Sure, go ahead.

Laura: You don't seem yourself lately, is there something bothering you?

Matthew: No, not really.. I mean, I don't really care anymore.

Laura: Don't care about what?

Matthew: About my life, I guess.

Laura: What would make you feel that way? Your making progress right?

Matthew: Yes, but all for what? I have no real life anyway. I never have.

Laura: Your still young Matthew and have your whole like ahead of you. How about your friends?

Matthew: I have had difficultly in forming lasting relationships. I am not close to my brother and my father left when I was only seven years old. My mom is all I really have and she is getting along in years.

Laura: Is that why you have always turned to food, for comfort?

Matthew: I guess you can say food has always been my friend.

Laura: There is nothing wrong with enjoying food as long as it does not become a health issue and dominate your life. I have a friend that has an eating disorder and attends a support group. It's a great place to share issues in your life that have driven you to over eating. Would you like to attend a meeting? I would be happy to go with you.

Matthew: I don't know Laura. I mean, I am not big on sharing my personal life with a bunch of strangers!

True Calling
Laura Marie Patterson

Laura: You do not have to share anything if you don't feel comfortable. The main reason is to listen to others explain their challenges and to know that you are not alone.

Matthew: Okay, I will try one meeting.

After discussing the benefits with my Care Manager of Matthew attending the over eaters support meeting, I was given the green light for us both to attend. The following Monday evening we attended the first over eaters support group meeting. It was hosted by the local church and was held in their large multipurpose room. There were between 30-40 people in attendance sitting in an informal semi-circle of chairs. We both quietly took our seats towards the back of the room just as the meeting began.

The guest speaker for the evening was a reasonably attractive middle aged woman that carried a healthy weight and a bubbly personality. She began by reading from a book that explained the philosophy of their twelve step program and what was expected from the members of the group. Much like any addiction support group, the focus was on recovery and maintaining abstinence from over eating. The core of the meeting consisted of testimonials from members that have had ninety days or more of abstinence. This included working with a sponsor on a daily basis and reporting what foods and the amount that was to be consumed. Each speaker would speak briefly about their struggle with food addiction and the emotional factors that have contributed to their need to over eat.

Matthew sat in silence and listened intently to each member share their experience, strength and hope. At one point all new comers were asked to identify and introduce themselves. Matthew did not raise his hand as he did not wish any attention from the group. I felt that when the time was right and he felt comfortable, Matthew would participate in the group. This being the first meeting it was enough for him just to attend.

When the meeting paused for the midway break, a gentleman approached Matthew and introduced himself as Charles. He appeared to be about Matthews age, tall and fairly thin. With a big smile on his face he repeated, "Matt, don't you recognize me? It's Charlie!"

Matthew: Charlie? I don't believe it! I have not seen you in years, and you look great!

Charlie: Yes, I have been going to the meetings now for about a year and half and I've lost over 200 pounds!

Matthew looked surprised to see his friend appearing so different than the last time he saw him. I could also tell that Matthew was embarrassed for Charlie to see him with even more weight than before. Matthew introduced me as his friend Laura that had suggested the meeting to him.

Charlie: Nice to meet you Laura. Matt and I go way back to our high school days. I had moved from the area for awhile and just returned a few years ago. Are you a member of the over eaters group also?

True Calling

Laura Marie Patterson

Laura: Nice to meet you too Charlie. No, I have a close friend Rebecca that is a member of the group and had also lost over 200 pounds. She had told me that coming here has helped her regain control of her life and of the great people that attend these meetings. I thought that Matthew might find inspiration and guidance here as well.

Charlie : Well, there is a fantastic group here that is very supportive of one another. When I started, I was unsure and had only attended a few meetings when I had stopped going. It was only when I returned and accepted a sponsor that I really began to see real progress and now I am a sponsor as well. Matt, I would like to sponsor you in the program. What do you think?

Matthew: Sure Charlie. What do I have to lose?

Charlie: Lots of weight for starters!

We all three laughed and I was excited and happy that Matthew was able to connect with an old friend and one that was willing to help him. After the meeting Matthew and Charlie exchanged phone numbers and Matthew told me of Charlie and his friendship while in school.

Matthew: Charlie and I where known as the "Boom-Boom Brothers" we were both pretty hefty and hung out together all the time. Charlie had similar family problems as his dad was an alcoholic and was abusive to him and his mother. We would share our tales of woe over a burger or two, or three..

Laura: It is easy to understand how you both would turn to eating as way of escaping your difficult family situations. After seeing Charlie again this evening, does it make you feel more hopeful about yourself?

Matthew: For one thing it was great to see Charlie again and that he is doing so well. He is going to call me tomorrow morning so we can start on my recovery program and talk about old times.

Laura: That is great Matthew! Charlie seems like a great guy and it will be good to have your old friend back in your life.

As promised the next morning Charlie called Matthew and they worked out a food plan. We were to measure 6oz of protein for each meal along with 12oz of vegetables. For breakfast he could have a whole grain fiber cereal along with 8oz of fruit. We continued our daily walks which we increased to several blocks around the neighborhood. Charlie would often visit Matthew during the weekends. Matthew would get out of the house for awhile as they rekindled their friendship.

Matthew continued to lose weight as he and Charlie continued the program and attending the support meetings twice weekly. After about six months of working with Matthew he announced that he would be moving out of his mothers house and that Charlie and he were to share a place together. By that time Matthew had lost over 100 pounds and was doing much better than when I first started working with him.

True Calling
Laura Marie Patterson

Charlie was a great influence and role model for Matthew and would continue to keep Matthew focused on his goals moving forward. I felt positive about Matthew's future and still came by to visit with his mother when I was in the area.

Betty told me that both her and Matthew were grateful for all I had done for him. I told her that it was Matthew's determination and her love for her son that made all the difference. I was truly blessed to have witnessed such a transformation and rebirth in one man's life.

True Calling
Laura Marie Patterson

Chapter 3   Matthew- Finding Comfort in Food

Resource Index

Appendix A: Building Trusting Relationships   158

Appendix F: Working with Family Members   182

Appendix C: Nutrition and Food Preparation   166

Related Chapters

Chapter 5: William - Building Trust   70

This page was left blank intentionally.

Chapter 4
Kathy – A Family in Turmoil

True Calling
Laura Marie Patterson

Chapter 4

Kathy - A Family in Turmoil

*O*n the weekends, I would occasionally accept relief assignments from my agency. One Sunday I was asked to fill in for the regular caregiver of a lady with multiple sclerosis. Her name was Kathy, a young and bright woman that began showing signs of the disease in her early 20s. Multiple sclerosis is devastating and progressive illness that affects the brain and spinal cord. In Kathy's case, the MS had progressed to the point were she was paralyzed from the shoulders down.

Her home was located in a nice quiet neighborhood and secluded from the street. As I drove down the driveway I could see a large ranch style home. After parking my car to the side of the garage, I walked up to the double red front doors and noticed a bright yellow note attached that read "Caregiver please come in. Kathy's room is at the end of the hallway, the last door on the right" I was surprised to find that Kathy was at home alone considering her restrictive disabilities.

The house was tastefully decorated and in neat order. As I reached the end of the hall, I announced my arrival at Kathy's door. "Hello, I'm Laura your caregiver for today"

Kathy: Come on in Laura.

As I opened the bedroom door, I saw Kathy with a pleasant smile as she laid in bed. I could see a bed tray across her lap that had several objects sitting on it.

Laura: Good Morning Kathy, are we alone in the house?

Kathy: Yes Laura, my brother and my sister in-law left about an hour ago. They should return before you leave this evening.

Laura: What if there would be an emergency and no one was at home to assist you?

Kathy: You see, I have this special pointing device on my tray that I can use in my mouth to press the speed dial buttons on this pad. I can call my brother's cell phone, 911 or several other numbers and then speak through the speaker phone. I can also control my T.V. remote using it as well.

Laura: It must take some practice to achieve the accuracy needed to do all of that?

Kathy: You learn as a matter of necessity. I have become very good at it.

Her voice was clear but labored as she spoke. I could tell that she had some difficulty using her lungs due to her advanced MS however, her words were articulate. I was profoundly moved by her resilience and could tell that she was a determined woman with a strong will to survive.

True Calling
Laura Marie Patterson

Laura: I am truly impressed by your ingenuity Kathy. You have a beautiful place here. Is this your brother's home?

Kathy: Actually, it belongs to both of us. After my parents were killed in a car accident, my brother and I were left this home and all the furnishings. That was almost seven years ago. I moved in with my brother and his wife about 3 years ago after my divorce.

Laura: I am so sorry to hear about your parents Kathy. So how long were you married?

Kathy: We were married just short of our 10th year anniversary and we have a son Billy. He will be 13 in a two weeks.

As Kathy continued to speak you could see that her smile was replaced by sadness as tears began to form.

Laura: Does your son live close by?

Kathy: He lives with my ex-husband across the bay. I have not seen him in almost six months but I do talk to him once or twice a week. I understand it's very hard on him seeing me in this condition, but I do miss my little boy.

Laura: It's good that your able to live here and have your brother and his wife's help.

Kathy: Well.. he really has no choice in the matter since I do own half this home. He now wishes to sell but I won't budge. They want to move up to Oregon and put me in a facility, but this is also my home and it's where I want to remain till my final day.

Laura: I can understand why you would rather wish to stay here. So your brother is not willing to wait until such time?

Kathy: Quite frankly Laura, my brother Dave is surprised I am still here. Even after the doctors told me that I would most likely not see my 30th birthday, I refused to believe it. I am now 32 years old and although I have very little use of my body, I still have my mind. My personal goal has been to see my son graduate high school. I may not make it, but I am not ready to give up yet. Being here in my parents home is a comfort to me. I grew up in this house and it gives me strength just being here.

Laura: You deserve peace and serenity especially during this challenging time in your life. I am sorry to hear of all the turmoil that your family is facing.

Kathy: Thank you Laura. I really did not intend on dumping all this on you, since you just have arrived. Please have a seat, relax and tell me about yourself.

After hearing of Kathy's intense situation, I knew that she needed and wanted a distraction. I began telling her about the circumstances that lead to becoming a caregiver and what a rewarding experience that it has been so far.

True Calling

Laura Marie Patterson

Laura: You know Kathy, if someone would have told me years ago that this is where I would be at this point of my life, I would have been hard pressed to believe them. Starting out as a musician playing guitar and then a software engineer has been a real transition however, I have to admit I do enjoy my work as challenging as it is at times.

Kathy: Oh, I would love to hear you play your guitar sometime. I just love music, it's one of the escapes that I have to enjoy. As you can see on the shelf, I have many CDs.

As I turned to the bookcase beside me, I could see the many CDs that were lined on the top shelf. As I began glancing through the titles, I noticed the varied artists and genres she had in her collection. There were a number of classical albums as well.

Laura: Sure Kathy. It would be my pleasure to play for you, but I am just filling in today and I am not sure if I will be back next week.

Kathy: I hope you can return next Sunday. My current weekend caregiver is very sweet but not very talkative. She is from Panama and her is English is not very good.

Laura: I see, possibility something can be worked out. I will call the office in the morning and see what I can do but for now is there anything that I can get for you?

Kathy: Yes, could you please get some juice for me? Use this cup on my tray. It may need to rinsed out and may I have a clean straw?

Laura: Certainly, I will be right back with your juice. Would you like something to eat as well?

Kathy: Just some juice for now Laura, thank you.

As I headed back down the hallway towards the kitchen, I admired the beautiful artwork that hung on the walls, before reaching the kitchen. I saw the family room to the right and noticed a table with picture frames arranged on top. There were many family photos but did not notice that Kathy's picture was included. I did see a photo of an older couple that must have been Kathy's parents along with some more recent wedding photos of another couple which I assumed were Kathy's brother Dave and his wife.

I turned away and continued into the large kitchen that looked to have been recently remodeled. As I began rinsing the cup in the sink, my mind wondered back to what Kathy had said about her son being so uncomfortable visiting her. I can't imagine the difficulty he must have had with first his mother's illness and then his parent's divorce. What could have caused the separation of the family at such an emotional and critical time? As a caregiver, it can be very difficult to distance yourself and not want to be involved with your clients personal matters, however, at the same time you are there to support your client emotionally and be a shoulder to cry on if need be.

I filled the glass with apple juice, grabbed a fresh straw from the cabinet and then headed back to Kathy's room. As I entered her room I noticed that she had turned on the T.V. and was watching an old movie.

Laura: Here you are Kathy, is apple juice okay?

True Calling

Laura Marie Patterson

Kathy: That is fine, thank you Laura.

Laura: What movie are you watching?

Kathy: Oh it's one of my all time favorites, Withering Heights with Laurence Olivier and Geraldine Fitzgerald. Have you ever seen it?

Laura: I have heard of the name, but can't remember what the movie was about. Was it not adopted from a famous novel?

Kathy: That's correct, it was written in the mid 1800s by Emily Bronte and is about love between two soul-mates, Cathy, a girl from a wealthy family, and Heathcliff, a gypsy boy without means. Cathy also cares for her neighbor Edgar which is worldly and refined. I don't want to give away more about the film and spoil it for you.

As we watched the movie together, I could tell that Kathy really enjoyed having my company. There were parts in the movie where Kathy would add a few comments, such as when Cathy chose Edgar over Heathcliff, "She is only making that decision based on what others would think if she married Healthcliff." and "Money does not make the man, it's love and loyalty that matters the most." I felt that Kathy's comments about the movie somewhat mirrored her own life. Had she also married her husband for the wrong reasons?

Laura: That was a great movie Kathy. Thank you for sharing it with me.

Kathy: Your welcome. I think it is like the 100th time I have seen this movie.

Laura: Do you mind if I ask you a personal question?

Kathy: No, not at all. My life is an open book.

Laura: What was behind your divorce? I mean, was there an issue of infidelity?

Kathy: Actually Laura it was a couple of things. When Steve and I first met, I was just ready to graduate from Cal State Berkeley with my BA in applied science. Steve on the other hand was working as a mechanic and had attended college but decided to drop out in his second year. We were introduced by a mutual friend and it was love at first sight. After dating for about 6 months we decided to get married, but there were conditions.

Laura: Conditions on you?

Kathy: Steve wanted to start his own shop so he could work for himself, but that also meant that I would have to put my masters degree on hold for awhile. I did not mind supporting his dream as long as I could go back and continue my studies after his business was established. A year later we were married and I began showing symptoms of MS. It was then, I began seeing a string of doctors, undergoing tests and treatments.

Laura: So how is Steve's business doing now?

True Calling
Laura Marie Patterson

Kathy: He has one of the biggest automotive repair shops in the East Bay and doing very well business wise. The issue Steve has now is his drinking and womanizing which is not a healthy environment for my son. I am not saying that he does not love our son or he is not a good father, he just has to get his priorities in order.

Laura: I am sorry how things turned out for you. Was your MS a determining factor in your divorce?

Kathy: He used it more as an excuse for his behavior. I understand the stress that my illness put in our marriage, but if he would have taken his vows seriously our family would have remained complete.

Later that afternoon, I assisted Kathy with her bathing. After removing her clothing, I transferred her to the wheelchair using a special device called a Hoyer Lift. I had some training using this piece of equipment both in my class and previously with another client. There was an open shower which was specially built to accommodate her wheelchair. Because Kathy could not help in anyway, it was fortunate that Kathy was a petite girl and weighed less than 100 pounds, so moving her was not to difficult for me.

Another necessary task was to assist Kathy with her bowel movements. Bowel dysfunction is common with multiple sclerosis and needs to be addressed aggressively with regular scheduling, fluid intake, suppositories and enemas. caregiving is providing the client with both emotional and physical care. This is an area where some caregivers will have issues. I had some experience assisting with bathing and toileting however, because of Kathy's condition she required a higher level of care. With each new case the caregiver adds to his or her training and experience.

Kathy's nutrition was also key to managing her symptoms and her longevity. Her diet was based on white meat, fish, fruit, vegetables, including vitamin supplements, in particular vitamin D3. Since Kathy did not have the use of her hands, I needed to provide her with feeding assistance. One important thing to remember is that the client needs to enjoy their meal. Allowing ample time for them to eat their meals slowly and in the order they wish adds to their enjoyment. Kathy's meal was prepared in advance, so all I needed to do was to warm the food for her.

About a half hour before my shift was to end, Kathy's brother and his wife returned. I could hear the front door close and the sound of footsteps as Dave approached Kathy's room..

Dave: Hello you must be Laura? I am Kathy's brother Dave and this is my wife Susan.

Laura: Nice to meet you both. Your sister and I had an enjoyable day. She is a wonderful person.

Susan: Did you find the meal I had prepared for Kathy in the refrigerator?

Laura: Yes, thank you. I also assisted Kathy with her shower this afternoon.

Kathy's brother Dave was a tall, well groomed man with a deep looming voice. Susan was an attractive and stylishly dressed woman. Both appeared to be in their mid to late 30's.

True Calling
Laura Marie Patterson

Kathy: I really enjoyed Laura's company today. I am hoping she can return next Sunday.

Dave: What's wrong with Maria? She seems to work well with you.

Kathy: Maria is sweet and does a great job, it's just that it is difficult for us to talk.

Dave: I see, well that depends on Laura's schedule.

Laura: My Sunday's are free at this point however, I will need to talk with my care manager first. I will call her tomorrow and see if something can be worked out.

Dave: Okay fine by me. Nice meeting you Laura and we may see you next week then.

After Dave and Susan left the room, I arranged some things for Kathy and we then said our goodbyes.

Laura: I hope I can see you again next week. Thank you for trusting and sharing with me.

Kathy: Thank you for all you have done for me today, and I am truly hoping I will see you next week.

I reached down to give Kathy a hug. I could tell that it was good for her to be able to talk out her feelings. As I turned to say goodbye, Kathy gave me a warm smile as she also said goodbye.

The next morning I stopped by my agency's office to speak with Joanne the agency's administrator. As I approached her office, I could see that she was on the phone. She waved to me as I took a seat just outside of her office. A few minutes later she ended her call and told me to come on in.

Joanne: Hi Laura, how are you?

Laura: I am doing great Joanne, however I do have something I need to speak with you about.

Joanne: Sure, have a seat. How may I help you?

Laura: On Sunday, I was called to cover for Maria's client Kathy and she has requested that I return next Sunday.

Joanne: I am sure it can be arranged. I will give Lisa, your care manager a call and pass on the request. Is there anything else I can do for you?

Laura: There are some family issues that Kathy told me about that is concerning me.

Joanne: Okay Laura, you are correct in bringing them to our attention. So what are the issues that Kathy is having?

I explained to Joanne the pending problem with Dave wanting to sell their home and of his plan to place Kathy in a facility against her will.

True Calling
Laura Marie Patterson

Joanne: I can understand your concern over Kathy's distress, but with family issues there is little intervention that we can provide other than in the case of client safety or abuse.

Laura: I feel like Kathy is just in need of someone she can talk to. She is a strong and determined woman in spite of her multiple sclerosis. She appreciates Maria, but there is a language barrier that makes personal conversations difficult between them.

Joanne: Sometimes we need to reassign our caregivers in the best interest of the clients needs. In this case, Kathy has formed a connection with you which is good. Just beware of client confidentiality with any personal information that she shares with you.

Laura: I completely understand. Kathy just needs a friend right now, someone she can talk to. Instead of replacing Maria on the weekends, could I possibly just work with Kathy on Sundays?

Joanne: Okay, I will see that it is arranged. Thanks Laura, and give my best to Kathy.

During the course of the week, my thoughts would often go back to Kathy. I wondered if her brother would postpone his plans on selling the house while Kathy is still living there and what about her son? I was hoping that he would visit her on his 13th birthday. All I can really do is to give Kathy a pleasant Sunday and hopefully a break from her stress and worry.

The following Sunday morning, I loaded my guitar into the car and headed to Kathy's for the day. I remembered her requesting that I play my guitar so I thought it would be a pleasant surprise for Kathy. As I approached the house I noticed her brothers truck was parked in the drive way and the garage door was open. I parked my car beside the garage and with my guitar in hand I headed towards the front door. Just as I rang the door bell I heard Dave call out to me from the garage. "Go on in Laura, Susan is in the kitchen." I thought before heading to Kathy's room I would let Susan know that I was there first. As I walked into the kitchen. I saw that Susan was chopping some vegetables in front of the sink.

Laura: Good morning Susan.

Susan: Oh.. hi Laura nice to see you again. Kathy has been looking forward to your visit all week long and you have brought your guitar with you, how nice!

Laura: Yes, I promised Kathy that I would play sometime for her.

Susan: I am so glad you could arrange your Sunday's to work with Kathy. She has been upset all this week since her ex husband had told her that he is taking their son Billy out of town the week of his birthday.

Laura: I know that Kathy was hoping he might visit her on his 13th birthday. I just can't understand why he feels it necessary to keep so much distance between Billy and his mother?

True Calling

Laura Marie Patterson

Susan: You see, the more that Kathy's MS impacted her ability to function normally the more distant her husband became. He feels the need to protect Billy from seeing his mother in such a way. Eventually Kathy moved back here to live with us. It was either move here or to a care facility.

Laura: When I was talking with Kathy last week she mentioned something about you and your husband selling the house and moving to Oregon?

Susan: Those plans have been it the works for the last couple of years. It's just that there is a job opportunity up in Portland that Dave is very interested in. I am originally from Portland and my parents are still living up there. Dave and I wish to start a family, so it makes sense for us to relocate up there.

Laura: I can understand why you two wish to make the move, it's just that Kathy does not want to spend her remaining life in a facility. She told me that being here in her parents home has given her peace and strength.

Susan: I know Laura. We have had long discussions with Kathy about this opportunity for us and for her need to be practical.

Laura: I'm sorry I do not wish to interfere with your family's business, it just that Kathy seemed so determined about staying here in her parent's home until the end. As a caregiver, I am here to support my clients emotionally, but there is a thin line that I can not cross. However, it does help to know the circumstances behind the situation.

Susan: Since Kathy seems to really like you, perhaps you can help her to understand and accept a change in her living arrangements?

Laura: It's not really my place to make those kind of suggestions to Kathy. Have you thought about bringing in a third party to council the family?

Susan: We have thought about that, but it's not a bad idea. Kathy is seeing us as the enemy and we are not. We love her and only want what's best for her.

Laura: I can see that Susan. Maybe in conversation I can suggest a meeting with a family counselor?

Susan: Thank you Laura. Dave and I would really appreciate anything you can do to help.

Laura: Okay, I will see what I can do. Are you and Dave leaving for the day?

Susan: Yes, we will be gone for the most of the day visiting friends so you will have plenty of time alone with Kathy.

I told Susan I would see them later and to have a nice day as I left the kitchen and headed down the hall to Kathy's room. I really felt sad for Kathy, especially the fact of not being able to be with her son on his birthday. I could see that Kathy's door was open as I reached her room.

True Calling
Laura Marie Patterson

Laura: Good morning Kathy

Kathy: Laura, I am so happy to see you!

Laura: I also brought my guitar with me today

Kathy: Yes, I can see that! I am looking forward to hearing you play for me.

The next hour was spent performing basic ADLs which means, "Activities of Daily Living". This includes bathing, dressing, mouth care and basic grooming. Dave and Susan had left shortly after I arrived, so again it was just Kathy and I alone in the house. Although Kathy was initially happy to see me, I could see the disappoint over missing her son's birthday as she tried her best to hide her emotions. When she is ready she will talk about it. What could I say to make her feel better? Sometimes just being there for someone is enough.

Laura: Now that we have you all cleaned up and pretty, are you ready for something to eat?

Kathy: No thank you Laura, I am not very hungry.

Laura: Okay, maybe after awhile then. How are you feeling today?

I could see Kathy's effort to hold back her tears as she told me of her husband's plans to take their son out of town on his birthday.

Kathy: When Steve called to tell me that he was taking Billy out of town next week, I asked if he could stop by here first so I could spend a little time with my son before they left. He said that they would be leaving early in the morning and there would not be an opportunity to stop by here first, since they are heading inland towards the lake. Steve did say he would call on their way so that I could speak with Billy.

Laura: That's good Kathy. You will be able to wish him happy Birthday then. You mentioned last week that it had been six months since you had last seen Billy? Do you mind my asking who's decision that was?

Kathy: When Steve and I first separated, it was very hard on Billy. He was only 10 years old at the time, and although I had been dealing with my MS most of his life, it really was not that obvious to him in the early stages. As the MS developed and I was restricted to a wheelchair, that is when things began to change. It was like Steve just pulled the plug on our marriage and felt the need to shelter Billy from the pain of seeing his mother fade away.

Laura: I am so sorry Kathy. That certainly is not fair to you or is it a good example for Billy to follow. Billy needs not to see your MS as barer to your relationship but as a unavoidable tragedy. He needs to learn to from your determination and strength to fight the disease. Have you spoken to anyone from social services about your visitation rights with Billy?

True Calling
Laura Marie Patterson

Kathy: Yes I have a few times, but when they interviewed Billy, he just told them that he does not really want to spend much time here with me because it's "boring with nothing to do." I can understand that a young boy would rather spend the time with his father.

Laura: Steve should be encouraging Billy to spend more time with you while he is able. There will come a time in his life when those memories of you will be treasured. Kathy, would you be open to talking about these issues with a third party?

Kathy: What do you mean?

Laura: About the issues between you and your brother and the relationship with your son. Maybe a family counselor could help?

Kathy: I don't know Laura, social services has not been much help with Billy in the past and I don't know how open my brother would be to the idea of someone sticking their nose in their business.

Laura: This is also about you Kathy and your needs. If, I could get your brother to agree to a visit from a family counselor, would you be willing to participate?

Kathy: Yes, I am always willing to discuss things, that has never been the problem.

Laura: Okay then, I will pass this request along to my Care Manager Lisa and she will follow up with you.

Kathy: Lisa was by on Wednesday to tell me that you would be available to work with me on Sundays. She is sweet person but seems very busy and distracted.

Laura: Care Managers have a very big responsibility to both the clients they serve and the caregivers that they support. I am sure that she had many appointments that day.

Kathy: I do appreciate all that you are doing in my behalf. I feel that I finally have someone on my side.

Laura: I do believe that everyone has your best interest at heart Kathy. I think it's more of an issue of mutual understanding. I am sure your family will benefit greatly with some professional intervention.

The rest of the day was spent enjoying music. I played my guitar for Kathy and we also listened to some of her CDs. Kathy also shared her photo albums with me. There were photos of Billy at different ages along with other family photos. I can only imagine how painful it must be for Kathy to look back at happier times, but instead she said that it gives her pause to smile. What a truly remarkable woman.

The next morning I left a message for Lisa to call me about Kathy's situation. Later that afternoon Lisa had returned my call..

Laura: Thanks Lisa for returning my call. Kathy's family is requesting a counselor. Could you give Susan, her sister-in-law a call with a possible referral?

True Calling
Laura Marie Patterson

Lisa: That's wonderful Laura! How did you get Kathy to agree to this?

Laura: It started with Susan asking if I could make the suggestion. In a conversation with Kathy, I asked if she would be open to the idea of a third party intervention.

Susan: I know of a great family therapist that probably would be willing to do a home visit. I will make the call and set the wheels in motion. Thanks Laura for your concern for Kathy and her family.

The following Sunday as I approached Kathy's room I could hear voices and laughter. As I entered the room I saw a young boy sitting on the edge of Kathy's bed holding a book. There was a big smile and a radiance on Kathy's face as she turned her head to greet me.

Kathy: Good morning Laura this is my son Billy!

Laura: Nice to meet you Billy and happy birthday! What are you two reading?

Billy: My mom bought this joke book for my birthday and it's so funny!

I could see the strong resemblance between Billy and his mother. At 13 he seemed a bit immature for his age. It was a heart warming sight to see Kathy and her son together.

Laura: Kathy, I am going to head to the kitchen and leave you two alone for awhile. Can I get you two anything?

Kathy: Thanks, I am fine right now Laura.

Billy: My Dad will be picking me up soon. We are going to have pizza for lunch.

Laura: Oh, that sounds yummy! I love pizza too. I will back in a while. You two continue to have fun. As I walked down the hallway towards the kitchen Susan walked out from one of the bedrooms.

Susan: Hello Laura. Did you meet Billy?

Laura: Yes, I am so happy the his father brought him over for a visit. What had changed his mind?

Susan: After you left last week, Kathy asked if I could stop by the bookstore and find a book for Billy. They used to love to read the comic section of the newspaper together and Kathy thought he might enjoy a joke book. Kathy called Steve and told him that she had a special birthday gift for Billy. They had a long discussion and the next thing I knew Steve changed his plans for the fishing trip and brought Billy by here for visit instead.

Laura: That's wonderful. I am so happy for the both of them!

Susan: Also, I would like to thank you for setting up the session with Frank Rogers the family therapist. We have an appointment with him next Tuesday evening, and he offered to come to our home.

True Calling
Laura Marie Patterson

Laura: Your welcome, but you also need to thank Lisa for the referral. I just brought your request to her attention. I am hoping that you can openly discuss the difficult issues along with Kathy and agree upon a mutual plan.

Susan: We really have Kathy's best interest in mind. I just hope that Kathy can understand our position.

Laura: I too am hoping for the best. Since Billy's father will be here soon to pick him up, I thought I would give them more time alone. I will be in the kitchen if she needs me.

Susan: Okay, thanks Laura.

I was washing a few dishes and preparing some fresh vegetables for the evening meal when I heard a car pull up in the driveway. Looking out the kitchen window I saw a nice sports car driven by a man. This must be Steve, Billy's father. I watched as he got out of his car and made his way to the front door. Steve appeared to be a nice looking man that was neatly dressed. I heard the front door open. Steve walked in and I met him in the hallway.

Steve: Hello you must be Laura?

Laura: Yes, and you must be Steve, Billy's father?

Steve: That's correct. I am here to pickup Billy. Is he in his mothers room?

Laura: Yes, they are reading the joke book that Kathy gave him for his birthday.

As Steve heading down the hall towards Kathy's bedroom, I returned to the kitchen to leave them to their privacy. I could hear the faint voices of Billy and his father in the background. About 5 minutes later Steve and Billy were heading for the front door. I emerged from the kitchen just in time to say goodbye.

Laura: Have a great lunch Billy and don't eat to much pizza!

Billy: Goodbye Laura

Laura: Nice meeting you Steve

Steve: Same here and take care.

As soon as the front door closed I headed to Kathy's room.

Laura: How are you doing Kathy? Looks like you two enjoyed your visit.

Kathy: It was so nice to laugh again with Billy. It has been so long since we have just hung out and had fun together.

Laura: I am so happy for you both and glad that Steve made the time to bring Billy on his birthday.

Kathy: When I talked to Steve last week, I told him something that you had told me last Sunday.

Laura: What was that?

True Calling

Laura Marie Patterson

Kathy: Simply that Billy needs to spend time with me now because those memories will stay with him for the rest of his life.

Laura: That was generally what I had told you but you said it so much better. Good for you Kathy!

That afternoon we watched another old movie. This one was one of my all time favorites too, Bringing Up Baby. This movie featured Katharine Hepburn and Cary Grant made in 1938. I asked Kathy why she enjoyed old movies so much?

Kathy: Back then things were safer, simpler and even sexier. These movies are entertaining without being overly violent or rude. I guess I watch these movies to escape the reality of my life. I have had a long time to come to terms with my MS and I have refused to be a whiner but a fighter instead. I know that ultimately the MS will win, but I will do my best to make every last day I have count.

The next week I received a call from the agency informing me that Kathy would soon be relocating but I will still be needed the following Sunday. I was grateful to have the opportunity to spend one last day with Kathy and to say goodbye.

When I arrived at Kathy's home on Sunday, I noticed a trailer parked beside the garage and the front door open. As I walked up to the door Dave was just coming out the door carrying a box.

Laura: Hi Dave, looks like your busy?

Dave: Yes, I am just carrying a box of Kathy's things out to the trailer. Have you heard the news that she is relocating?

Laura: I received a call from Lisa last week and she told me Kathy would be moving soon and this was to be my last Sunday.

Dave: I will let Kathy fill you in on the details. I am just glad she is willing. In matter of fact, she is actually excited about it.

Laura: That's great news Dave! Can't wait to hear more about it from Kathy. I will talk to you later then.

As I entered Kathy's room I could see that the packing was indeed underway. There were several boxes already stacked in the corner of her room.

Laura: Good morning Kathy. Looks like your already busy packing. Where are you moving to?

Kathy: Hi Laura. I am moving across the bay just a couple of miles from Steve and Billy. It's actually a beautiful facility and I will have my own room with 24 hour care. Best of all, I will be close to Billy so that we can spend more time together.

Laura: That sounds wonderful! I am so glad you were able to work things out with your family. Obviously the meeting with the family counselor went well?

Kathy: Yes, Frank was just great. He was able to bring our family together so we could understand each others needs. I am going to miss this place, but I also realize that it is important to be close to Billy so that he has the opportunity to see me more often. Dave and Susan also need to move on with their lives as well.

True Calling
Laura Marie Patterson

Laura: Well, I certainly am going to miss you Kathy. You are a very brave and intelligent woman and it has been a real pleasure to spend time with you.

Kathy: Same here. It has been wonderful to have a friend to share my feelings and emotions with. Thank you Laura for being here and everything that you have done to help me and my family.

Laura: Your most welcome, and speaking of help, do you need some assistance with packing some more of your things?

Kathy: It would be great if you could help me dig through my closets.

We spent the most of the day sorting, folding and packing the clothing she wished to bring with her. At the end of the day I reached down to hug her as we both said our goodbyes. She just looked up and smiled brightly at me as I turned and left the room. I have never forgotten Kathy or her amazing spirit. The rewards we receive as caregivers does not arrive in an envelope at the end of each week. It is the special people that we help and the life lessons that we learn that are priceless.

Chapter 4   Kathy – A Family in Turmoil

Related Resources

Appendix A: Building Trusting Relationships   158

Appendix C: Nutrition and Food Preparation   166

Appendix F: Working with Family Members   182

Appendix E: Exercise and Social Activities   176

Related Chapters

Chapter 6: Francis - Finding Closure   102

Chapter 7: Sam - His Strong Will to Live   132

This page was left blank intentionally.

Chapter 5
William – Building Trust

Chapter 5

William - Building Trust

I have received a new and challenging assignment concerning a male client with advanced Parkinson's disease. As Lisa my care manager explained to me, the agency had sent a couple other caregivers for this case but the client was not cooperative and eventually refused their services. Lisa felt because of my previous experience with difficult clients that I may be successful with him.

William was a 58 year old man living in a large home with both his 34 year old daughter and elderly mother which had terminal cancer. His mother Ruth had hospice care so my assignment would be concerning William only. His daughter Tammy was single and working part-time as a secretary for her church. Lisa also advised that Tammy was very protective of both her father and grandmother which is understandable. This combination of Tammy's protectiveness and her father's lack of cooperation with caregivers could prove challenging.

I was told that I would be needed from 8:00am to 2:00pm Monday through Friday to assist with William's ADLs and work with him on his exercise therapies. I was the start this case the following morning.

The clients address was in an exclusive neighborhood on the otherside of town. As I arrived at their address there was an iron gate that crossed their wide driveway. I pressed the intercom button to announce my arrival. A woman's voice answered, "Hello, may I help you?"

"Hello. I am Laura your new caregiver sent by the agency"

"Hello Laura. Drive up to the front of the house and please park on the left side of the driveway"

"Okay, thank you!"

The sound of the chain and gears were heard as the gate slowly swung open. As I pulled up into the driveway and parked my car, the side door opened and young woman walked out to greet me.

"Hello, I am Tammy. How are today Laura?"

Laura: I am doing fine thank you. It's nice to meet you Tammy.

Tammy: Please come in Laura, I want to introduce you to my father.

I followed Tammy into the house, through the kitchen and into the family room where her father was sitting on the couch watching T.V.

Tammy: Dad this is Laura, the new caregiver the agency has sent to help you.

Her father just stared straight ahead ignoring my presence. His hands were trembling in his lap, a symptom of his progressing Parkinson's disease. He appeared thin, frail and older than his 58 years.

"Hello William, nice to meet you and I am looking forward to working with you."

True Calling
Laura Marie Patterson

Still no response from William as he continued intently watching his show on television.

"Would you care for a cup of coffee or tea while we have a little chat?"

"Sure Tammy, tea sounds wonderful."

I followed Tammy into the kitchen as she filled the kettle with water and turned on the stove to prepare our tea.

Tammy: So Laura, how long have you been caregiving?

Laura: About three years now. Prior to caregiving, I worked with computers for about 15 years.

Tammy: caregiving is quite a departure from computer work. Why the change in careers?

Laura: It was more a matter of necessity than anything else. The company I was contracted with in Hawaii was sold. I relocated to the bay area in search of employment but found few opportunities because of the dot com crash. I took a class for caregiving in hopes of landing a temporary position until things pick up in the computer field. After caregiving for awhile I found it so personally rewarding that I wanted to continue.

Tammy: That's very interesting Laura. You have a real challenge on your hands with my Father. He is a sweet guy but he can also be very stubborn at times.

Laura: I understand the worst approach a caregiver can take with a client such as your father is to be overly aggressive. The more you push a client for cooperation. the more resistance you may create. I will take things slow with your father and hopefully in time he will become comfortable with my assistance.

Tammy: Okay, thank you Laura. I really appreciate your willingness to work with my father. Let me give you a little more background. We lost my mother 8 years ago to breast cancer. At that time my father had not yet been diagnosed with Parkinson's. My dad has always been a hard worker and a strong independent man. After my mother passed, my dad had a very difficult time. It was the following year that he began to show signs of Parkinson's. I moved back home a couple of years ago to help my father and to assist with my grandmother which had also taken ill about the same time.

Laura: It must have been very difficult for you these last few years being a caregiver to family members, it is very hard both physically and emotionally.

Tammy: Yes, it has occupied most of my time. You see, I also work for my church in the office in the mornings. That is why I need your help, as I can't be in two places at one time.

Laura: I am more than happy to be here for you and help in any way I possibly can. How about your grandmother? Does she have a caregiver while your away?

True Calling
Laura Marie Patterson

Tammy: Hospice comes in the mornings to bathe and change her clothing. Also their is a nurse that visits twice a week. I would just appreciate that you check in on her when she is alone. I know you were only sent here to assist with my father but she will not need any extra care.

Laura: Sure, no problem. What hours will you be away?

Tammy: I will be leaving shortly after you arrive and I generally return about 2PM unless I need to stop at the market. I will call you if I am going to be late.

Tammy showed me around the house and explained what her father ate for breakfast and lunch. We also went over the recommended exercises that I would be encouraging her father to perform daily. This including short walks up the street and back and squeezing a red rubber ball in his hands to maintain his grip. She warned that her father liked watching television over doing his exercises so I will need to encourage him as much as possible.

Tammy: Okay Laura, I will leave you alone now while I go to work. If you have any questions or if there is a problem I can be reached on my cellphone. My number is on the refrigerator.

Laura: Thanks Tammy. We will be just fine and I will call if you I need anything.

After Tammy left for work I went to the family room where William was still watching television. He continued to ignore my presence as I sat quietly across from him on the other couch. We both sat in silence for about 1/2 hour as William finished watching his news show. Suddenly, he picked up the remote to turn off the television, his hands were trembling as he fumbled with the buttons. I wanted to help him but decided because of his independent nature, it would be best to allow him to do it for himself.

He slowly stood up from the couch and walked out to the hallway and towards the bathroom. I watched him as he entered the bathroom leaving the door slightly cracked open. Respecting Williams privacy, I stood just outside the door to listen for any assistance that he may need. A few minutes later, I could hear the water running at the sink as I opened the door just a bit more as to observe his activity. Although his actions were slow and his hands were shaking, William was able to wash his hands and face. When it came to brushing his teeth, that appeared to be more of a challenge for him. Perhaps a battery operated tooth brush might be a little easier and more effective for him?

After William finished washing and brushing his teeth he opened the door the rest of the way. I stood to one side and allowed him to continue down the hallway towards his room. I followed behind him but not too closely as he entered his bedroom. His clothes was neatly laid out on the bed. Tammy must have done this before I arrived. Again, I just stood outside his door in case he needed my help. I watched as he was able to sit on the edge of the bed and drop his pajama bottoms to the floor. He then lifted on leg at a time and slowly stepped out of them. He continued undressing as he fumbled with the rather large buttons of his pajama shirt. He was able to unbutton each one in order. Then he pulled one arm at a time from the sleeves as he removed his shirt.

True Calling
Laura Marie Patterson

Dressing was not as easy of a task for William as he attempted to pull his t-shirt over his head. At this point I knew it was time for me to assist him with his dressing. I walked into the room and stood beside him as I helped guide his head and then his arms through the openings of his t-shirt. Once that was accomplished then William was able to pull his t-shirt off on his own. We repeated the similar process as he put on his pants and then his shirt. I took his socks from the top of the dresser and rolled each one on his feet as he sat in silence and reluctantly accepted my assistance.

After William was dressed he headed back towards living room, sat down on the couch and returned to watching his show. All of this still without saying a single word. While William was in the living room occupied with his show, I thought I would look in on William's mother.

Ruth's bedroom was located at the other end of the house. Making my way through the kitchen and down the west end hall I could hear the sound of a television or radio coming from the back bedroom. As I approached her room, the door was open and there laid a frail elderly woman in bed. Next to her bed sitting on the night table was a tape player. As I stood at the entry of her door, I could hear the voice of a woman that sounded like she was reading a book. William's mother's eyes were closed as if she was asleep.

Just as I was ready to turn to leave as not to disturb her, I saw her eyes open. She noticed me standing in the door way as she reached for the button on the tape player. With the sound of the player muted, I introduced myself. "Hello, I am sorry to disturb you. My name is Laura, I am your son's new caregiver."

A weak and shaky voice replied, "Hello dear, my name is Ruth. nice to meet you."

Laura: Your grand daughter Tammy asked if I would check in on you. Is there anything that you need?

Ruth: Could you please fill my water pitcher and put a few ice cubes in for me?

Laura: Sure. May I ask what you are listening to?

Ruth: I am listening to books on tape. My eye sight is not so good anymore so the library sends me these books on tape. Have you ever read The Scarlet Letter?

Laura: I have heard of that book but never had the opportunity to read it. How nice that you can have these classic books provided to you in audio form. I will be right back with your water.

I headed to the kitchen to fill Ruth's water pitcher and on the way I checked on William, there he sat in the same position watching his show. (After I return from bringing Ruth's water pitcher filled, I will see if I can interest William in doing his exercises.)

As I carried the water pitcher back to Ruth's room, I noticed some photos that lined the hallway walls. One in particular caught my eye of a lovely dancer. The photo must have been taken many years ago, possibly during the 1930's.

Laura: Here you are Ruth. Can I fill your glass for you?

True Calling
Laura Marie Patterson

Ruth: Yes, please. Thank you.

Laura: Your welcome. I had noticed a beautiful photo of a dancer in the hall. Is that of a family member?

Ruth: Yes, actually that is a photo of myself when I was a professional dancer many years ago.

Laura: Oh my! How wonderful! You looked so graceful in that picture. Did you dance in the theater?

Ruth: I was one of the last Ziegfeld Follies Girls. We performed in films and in several Broadway productions. It was an exciting life and I have some great memories.

Laura: Sounds like you had a wonderful life. I would love to hear more about your career sometime when your feeling up to it. I was just thinking about working with your son on his exercises. He has not said anything to me yet, but I did help him get dressed this morning. I am just taking it slow right now and giving him his space.

Ruth: William is a good man. It's just he has always been independent and he does not easily accept help. Just have some patience with him, okay?

Laura: No problem. I will just give him time to get use to my presence. Perhaps he will be willing to take a short walk with me?

Ruth: Good idea. Don't ask him, just tell him it's time for his walk and see if he will just follow you out.

Laura: Okay. Thanks for the tip. I will be back later to check on you. Very nice meeting you Ruth.

Ruth: You also Laura and good luck with my son.

I headed back to the living room to hopefully get William to take his walk. Still intently watching the television, I sat next to him on the couch. "What are you watching William?" Still no response.

"It's nice out today. Would you like to go for a short walk to show me the neighborhood?"

He turned and looked at me with a half smile, then nodded his head as to say yes. "Great! since you know your way around I will just follow your lead." William slowly rose from the couch and headed toward the door with a slow shuffle.

I followed him out the door just two paces behind him. With his hands dangling beside him, he was well balanced on his feet. We walked up the driveway and then turned right walking down the sidewalk towards the end of the street. I slowly moved closer to William as I was now walking beside him. "Nice neighborhood you have here." William looked over and just nodded him head in agreement. We continued down to the end of the sidewalk until we were facing the large house at the end of the street. William just stood quietly looking at the trees that lined the long driveway to the house.

"These homes are beautiful William. Do you know who lives in this house we are now approaching with all the different colored rose bushes in their garden?"

True Calling
Laura Marie Patterson

In a low and muffled voice he answered.. "Doctor Steward."

Laura: I see.. are you two friends?

William: No, just know him and his wife

He then abruptly turned and headed back down the sidewalk. I was smiling as I followed behind him knowing that he had finally communicated with me. A small conversation for sure, but it was an important first step. We slowly made our way back to his home, this time walking down a small path on the other side of the house. As we made our way to the backyard, I noticed a wire fence that enclosed a small garden. I stood by and watched as William grabbed hold of a watering can that appeared to be filled with water as he struggled to lift it. I walked over and helped by holding the can from the bottom so that he could carry the can by the handle. We both moved in tandem walking side by side with the watering can to the garden area. I let William guide the direction as we watered each of the plants.

Laura: Did you plant this garden yourself?

William: My daughter did. I just water them.

Laura: That's a great activity for you William. Maybe after we finish with the watering, perhaps we can work on some strengthening exercises for your hands? That will help you lift your water can more easily.

William did not say anything and just nodded his head as in agreement. After watering the garden we entered the house through the back kitchen door. Once in the kitchen, William washed his hands in the sink and I followed by washing my hands too.

Laura: Would you like something to eat?

William: There is some fruit in the refrigerator.

Laura: Okay, why don't you go have a seat in the living room and I will cut up some fruit and bring some in to you?

William in his predictable fashion, nodded his head and shuffled to the living room. After bringing his fruit to him, I decided to once again check in on Ruth. As I approached her room this time, I did not hear the sound of her audio book playing. I looked into her room and saw that she was soundly sleeping. I walked away quietly as not to disturb her.

As I re-entered the living room, I saw that William was eating the fruit that I had prepared for him as he was back to his favorite past-time watching the television. I left him alone as I returned to the kitchen to make a phone call to Tammy. I dialed the number that she had written down for me. After a couple of rings she answered.

"Hello, Our Savior's Church.. this is Tammy, how may I help you?"

"Hello Tammy, this is Laura"

"Laura is everything alright?"

True Calling
Laura Marie Patterson

"Yes, just fine. I had just checked in on your grandmother and she is comfortably sleeping. We had a nice little chat earlier. She is a charming woman. Your father and I just returned from a walk and then watered the garden. He is having some fruit."

Tammy: So how are you two getting along?

Laura: It was a little slow at first, but your father is a real nice man and I feel as if I am slowly building his trust.

Tammy: That is wonderful Laura!

Laura: I was thinking about attempting some of his exercises with him.

Tammy: That would be great if you could get him to work with you. His squeeze ball and other exercise items are located in the cabinet below the T.V. Stand. There is an instruction sheet also that will explain the exercises and their recommended repetitions.

Laura: Okay, thank you. I am hoping that I can work on a daily routine with your dad that he will become comfortable with. I have found that is the best way for clients to be consistent with their exercises. In your fathers case, even more so in having trust with his caregiver.

Tammy: I have been praying for someone that can help my father. Laura, you seem to be that person. Thank you so very much!

Laura: Your welcome and I will do my best to work with your father to gain his confidence. I will see you later then.. goodbye.

I returned to the family room and opened the cabinet door below the television. I removed a box that contained a red rubber ball, an elastic exerciser and small hand-held weight. I also noticed a folded set of papers which outlined the various exercise routines and their duration along with a sheet for recording each days activity.

As I was going through the box, I could see that Williams attention was now focused on what I was doing. As I looked up, we made eye contact and I suggested to William while pulling out his red sponge ball and squeezing it in my hand, that we try doing some strengthening exercises.

Laura: This actually feels pretty good!

William did not answer.

"Here, catch!"

I tossed the ball underhanded towards William and in surprise he caught it!

I replied, "Good catch William!", as to encourage him to continue.

He then tossed it back to me. I recognized that a game had just began, so I squeezed the ball again and then tossed it back to him. This time before William tossed back the ball he squeezed it first. Each time the ball was tossed it was squeezed a few more times. The contest was to see how many times each of us could squeeze the ball before tossing it to the other. We then continued the game alternating hands every other toss.

True Calling
Laura Marie Patterson

I discovered the best way to work with William was to suggest rather than insist. Allowing a client to control their own activities independent of the caregivers guidance is preferred. William had always been a leader so following direction was not easy for him. This appeared to be a comfortable middle ground for William.

In the days that followed I had developed a routine with William. At exactly 8:10 after my arrival in the morning, William would head towards the bathroom where he would shower, shave and brush his teeth under my supervision. He would do well only needing minimal assistance at times. Then it was to his room where I would assist him with dressing for the day. Tammy would have his clothes ready for the day neatly laying across the chair, his shoes and socks placed in front of the chair. After William was dressed, he would head to the living room turning on the television to watch the morning news while I would be in the kitchen preparing his breakfast. Once breakfast was prepared and on the table I would just walk to living room entry and simply say, "it's ready!" William would then slowly rise from the couch and shuffle his way to the breakfast table where his breakfast and morning medication would be arranged on the table in the same way each morning. It is important for certain clients with memory or confusion issues to have routine in daily activities and to arrange items that they use each day in the same way.

While William would be having his breakfast I would head to his mother's room and check in on her. Generally the hospice nurse would arrive by 10:00am and Ruth would have her breakfast before Tammy left for work in the morning. As I approached her room I could hear the familiar sound of the narrator reading the book that she was listening to that day. Ruth was slightly propped up in bed as I opened her door. As soon as my presence was noticed she would press the pause button on the long cord leading to the tape player next to her bed.

Ruth: Good morning Laura.

Laura: Good morning to you too, and how are you feeling today?

Ruth: Not to well. I feel like my time on the earth is coming to a close and I am not feeling at peace with my granddaughter.

As Ruth spoke those words I could tell by the worried look on her face that she was consumed by despair over some unresolved issue with Tammy.

Laura: May I ask why you feel this way towards your granddaughter?

Ruth: She means well, and I do love her with all my heart, but she is always pushing her religious beliefs on me. Understand Laura, I have never been a very religious woman not to say I am not spiritual, but I have my own beliefs. Tammy feels that if I don't convert to her church beliefs that I will not be saved and go to heaven. Each morning she comes in my room, brings my breakfast and then begins the same old sermon.

True Calling

Laura Marie Patterson

Laura: Have you told her how you feel?

Ruth: We had a discussion awhile back and I did explain the way I felt. That I believe in a higher power and it is the good that you do in this life that is rewarded in your next life. I believe that we all return to earth again after we have passed. It's the experience that we gain over many lifetimes that makes each person unique, spiritually aware and in harmony with the universe.

Laura: That is a very interesting way at looking at life and our purpose on earth. There are so many different religions in the world and I feel that it is each individuals right to choose what beliefs that are best for him or her. The important thing is that your a good person and treat others with respect. I am sorry to hear that Tammy feels the need to convert your beliefs and that it is causing you such distress.

Ruth: I usually let it go in one ear and out the next but as I get closer to the end she feels the need as she puts it, "to save me from damnation and redeem my soul."

Laura: Some churches believe that the more non believers you save the more salvation you receive. There is nothing wrong in believing in your own religious views, but it's not really fair to insist on changing others beliefs especially when that person has lead a good spiritual life with pure intentions such as yourself.

Ruth: My late husband was a non believer in anything beyond the physical world. I believe in reincarnation and he believed that once your gone that is pretty much it. We would have discussions and sometimes debates, but we would always respect each others point of view. We were married for 56 wonderful years before he passed 3 years ago.

Laura: I am sorry that you have lost your husband but it sounds as if you had great harmony in your marriage.

Ruth: Yes, and it was meeting Russ that changed the direction of my life away from show business and towards a more traditional life as a wife and mother. I guess you could say I have had the best of both worlds and have no regrets in my decisions.

Laura: I am glad you are satisfied with the life that you had lived. Many people have unfulfilled dreams when they reach the end of their lives.

Ruth: I have no regrets, just the need to resolve this issue with my granddaughter Tammy. At times I feel I should just give in and let her believe that I have been saved in her way, but I don't know that I can really do that with a clear conscious.

Laura: Just know that I will be here for you to talk with whenever you feel the need to discuss your feelings, okay?

Ruth: Thank you Laura. It means a lot to me that you understand how I feel.

True Calling
Laura Marie Patterson

Laura: I do understand and I will talk to you later. Is there anything I can get for you before returning to your son?

Ruth: I am fine for now, thanks Laura.

As I headed back to the kitchen to check in on William, I could not help but carry the emotions expressed by Ruth in her frustration with her grand daughter. Certainly Tammy's love for her grandmother along with her commitment to her church has prompted the urgency to save her grandmother. I just hope that a mutual understanding can be reached so that Ruth can find peace in her final days.

William had finished his breakfast and was now back to watching the news on television. As I was cleaning up the breakfast dishes, I began to slowly formulate a plan that might bring Tammy and her grandmother to equal terms. However, it would require some intervention on my part. If only, Tammy could see herself through her own eyes?

The next morning I intentionally arrived a little early as to have the opportunity to talk with Tammy a few minutes before she left for work. As I tapped on the back door, Tammy peeked through the kitchen curtains to see who was . As she opened the door I greeted her with a big smile.

Laura: I hope my arriving early this morning is not disturbing you?

Tammy: No Laura, not at all. I was just having the rest of my coffee. Would you like some?

Laura: Yes thank you, that sounds wonderful. I was hoping we could talk for a few minutes?

Tammy: Certainly, is there a problem with my father?

Laura: No, William is fine. This is a personal problem that I am having that I thought you may help with.

Tammy: Sure Laura, I will try to help if I can. What is it concerning?

Laura: It's about my sister. I am afraid that she is making a bad decision and I am not sure what I should say or do about it. In a way it is none of my business, but on the other hand I am worried how this will play out with the rest of my family, along with my mother.

Tammy: I see. When it comes to family it can be a delicate situation. How old is your sister?

Laura: She is five years younger than me, has never been married and lives alone. Recently, she has become involved with a religious group that I know my mother would not approve of. You see Tammy, we were all raised strict Catholics and my sister joining this church could have bad consequences for my sister's relationship with our mother.

Tammy: Do you mind my asking what religious group your sister is considering joining?

True Calling
Laura Marie Patterson

Laura: I believe it is the Baptist church. It's not that she is joining a cult or something, it's just that my mother is such a strong believer in the Catholic ways that she will be worried for my sister's spiritual well being.

Tammy: What your mother needs to understand is a belief in God is the most important thing. What church you attend does not matter in the eyes of the lord, it's that you worship him in congregation and live your life according to the bible.

Laura: So Tammy.. when you say the bible, do you mean the bible of your personal beliefs?

Tammy: There is only one bible.

Laura: Yes, I agree. In my opinion, it's not the bible that you read, it's how you live your life. My sister is a good person so I will not judge her on which church she attends or whether she chooses to believe the same as the rest of our family, only that she is spiritually aware and treats others with respect.

Tammy: As long as your sister accepts Jesus Christ as her savior she will be saved and go to heaven. So it does not matter which church she attends.

Laura: Maybe the best way to put it to my mother would be the church of my sister's choosing is the God of her understanding?

Tammy: I think that would be a good way to present it to your mother, although I still believe that there is only one true bible and only one God.

Laura: I do respect your beliefs Tammy. Don't you feel that respecting someone's individual beliefs are important?

Tammy: Yes I do. Can I ask you a question Laura?

Laura: Sure.

Tammy: Has my grandmother been talking with you?

Laura: Yes, she has mentioned your discussion about her personal beliefs and it is a bit distressing for her.

Tammy: She has never expressed that feeling to me. I love my grandmother and want to make sure that she joins the rest of our family in heaven.

Laura: When you say the "rest of your family", does this include your grandfather too?

Tammy's face turned very serious and the tone of her voice changed as she continued..

Tammy: Look Laura, this is really none of your business in the first place! You were brought in here to take care of my father and look in on my grandmother and not to interfere in my relationship with my family!

True Calling
Laura Marie Patterson

Laura: I am sorry Tammy. It was not my intention to interfere in your family's business. I think your grandmother is a very sweet person and loves you with all of her heart. Speaking with me was her way of reaching out to you. All I am asking is to understand that she has a right to her own beliefs. What she needs the most from you now is your love and support in her final days.

Tammy's face now turned from serious to sad as the tears begin to form in her eyes.

Tammy: Laura, I am sorry. I did not mean to get angry with you. I just had no idea that my grandmother was so upset by my attempts to save her. I remember my grandfather when I was a little girl would sit me on his lap and explain how the earth came to be. He said it was formed by a giant explosion that formed all the planets and the space that we know as our universe. It scared and confused me because I was taught that everything was created by God in six days and on the seventh day he rested. Several years later I spoke to my pastor about what my grandfather had said. He told me that some do not believe there is a God and attempted to explain their existence with science. It was very difficult for me to accept my grandfather did not believe the same as the rest of the family. I loved my grandfather just the same and prayed for him, but he never changed his view.

Laura: Well Tammy, you said it best. You loved your grandfather anyway in spite of his different beliefs. Your grandmother only wants peace, comfort and your love. I hope that you both can put your religious differences aside and spend some quality time together with the days that she has remaining.

92

Tammy: Thank you Laura. I understand what you are saying and I will pray for the lord's guidance.

Laura: Your welcome, Tammy. I need to get started with your father as I know you need to get to work yourself.

Tammy: Okay, I will see you this afternoon.

The rest of the day was filled with thoughts of Tammy and her grandmother. I knew I was walking a gray line with my intervention, but on the other hand I felt compelled to at least bring awareness to Tammy about her grandmother's feelings. When I first started caregiving I did not realize the situations and family dynamics that a caregiver could encounter. In most cases, it is best not to get involved with your client's family matters. However, from my past experiences a certain amount of involvement can bring about positive results. It's best to go with your heart. If you are unsure seek the advise of a superior or other impartial person for their opinion and guidance.

On Monday morning, I returned to work and as I began my turn into their driveway to park, I noticed my spot was already taken by an unknown vehicle. I gently backed out of the driveway and parked my car in an empty spot across the street. As I made my way towards the house, I wondered who's car was parked in the driveway?

I rang the door bell and was shortly greeted by an unfamiliar woman.

"Hello I'm Laura, William's caregiver."

"Yes Laura. I am Nancy, Ruth's niece. Please come in."

Laura: Is everything okay? How is William and Ruth?

True Calling
Laura Marie Patterson

Nancy: William is fine, but my aunt has become very weak. The hospice nurse is with her now. I got a call over the weekend that my aunt had taken a turn for the worst so I drove up from Fresno to be with her.

Laura: I am so sorry to hear this. Ruth is very sweet and we have become close during the time I have cared for her son. Where is William?

Nancy: He is in his room. He is very upset and we have not been able to get him to come out since yesterday afternoon. He knows the end is near for his mother.

Laura: Thank you for the update Nancy, and nice to meet you. I will go and check on William. Please tell Tammy I am here.

Nancy: Sure Laura, and nice to meet you too.

As I headed down the hallway towards William's room, I could hear several voices coming from the dining room where the family was gathered. William's door was partially opened as I approached his room.

"William, it's Laura. Can I come in?"

From inside his room I could hear a grumbled "yes." As I opened the door the rest of the way, there sat William on the edge of the bed. William's head hung low to his chest supported up by the palms of his hands, he lifted his head as to greet me with his eyes, when I asked him if he was okay?

94

With no reply to my question, William turned his head away from me and returned to his original position before I entered his room.

"I am sorry about your mother William and understand how you must feel. Maybe if you came out and had something to eat you would feel better?"

Still, no response from William, I continued speaking letting him know that his family was very concerned about him and loved him very much.

Suddenly, without a word, William slowly stood up. I immediately turned around, praying that William would follow my steps. As I walked down the hallway, I was relieved to hear the shuffle of Williams feet behind me, as we made our way into the dining room.

There sat his family around the dining room table waiting for William's arrival, as my eyes made contact with William's daughter Tammy, she started to introduce me to each member of the family from left to right.

Tammy: Hi Laura, let me introduce you to some of my family. Laura is William's caregiver. She has been a great help with both dad and grandma over the last three months. Laura, this is my uncle Thomas, his wife Emily and my cousins Mike and Shirley. You have already met my cousin Nancy at the door.

Just as Tammy was finished making introductions, William stepped around the corner and entered the room.

True Calling

Laura Marie Patterson

Tammy: Hi dad! Come sit next to me.

William continued his shuffle over to where Tammy had pulled out a chair for her father.

Laura: I am going to fix something for William to eat. Can I get something for anyone?

Tammy: I think we are all fine Laura, thanks. There is some left over fruit cut up in the refrigerator that you can serve my dad.

Laura: Okay, thanks Tammy.

From the kitchen I could hear Tammy talking to her father.

Tammy: Dad, Grandma has been asking for you. As soon as the nurse is finished with her we will go in to see her.

I finished putting together a plate for William and headed back to the dining room.

Laura: Here you are William, have something to eat.

Tammy: Thanks Laura. Have a seat while we wait for the nurse to finish. Grandma was asking about you yesterday. She will be glad that you are here.

Just as Tammy finished speaking the nurse came into the dining room.

"Ruth is very weak but awake. You can go in now, however I suggest just a few at a time."

Tammy: Dad let's go see grandma.

Tammy and her father left for Ruth's room and I remained at the table with the others.

Nancy: Laura, how long have you been doing this kind of work?

Laura: About three years now. I used to work in the computer field, but after taking my first caregiving job I figured it was a time for a change. I do enjoy my work, but it is times like these that are very difficult.

Nancy: Tammy tells me that you have done wonders with William and he seems to respond well to you. I guess you either have the knack or you don't.

Laura: I would not say it's a knack more than patience. It takes time to build trust with a client and in William's case he was not very receptive to caregivers in general. We took baby steps together and after awhile we understood one another. I guess that is why I find caregiver challenging and rewarding.

Shortly after, Tammy came back while William remained in his mother's room.

Tammy: I left dad alone to be with grandma for awhile. I really don't think she has much time left. She told me to thank everyone for coming and wants me to send Laura in next.

Laura: How is your father handling things now?

True Calling
Laura Marie Patterson

Tammy: About as well as could be expected. He was always very close to grandma.

Laura: I understand how difficult this must be for him and all of you.

Tammy: We all knew this day would come, it was just a matter of time.

William returned to the dining room and took his seat. He said nothing as he stared straight ahead as if no one else was in the room.

Laura: I guess it's my turn now. I will be back shortly.

Tammy: It's okay, take all the time you need.

As I entered Ruth's room, I could not help but remember the very first day I met her and her bright cheerful smile. Now she laid in bed with her eyes barely open and with an expressionless face. I sat down next to the bed close to her. As she realized my presence and began to speak..

"Laura, I am glad you are here. I wanted to tell you something."

"Yes, Ruthie."

Ruth: I wanted to thank you for taking such good care of my son. He told me that he likes you. Also, I know you that you had spoken to my granddaughter about what I had told you.

Laura: I am sorry Ruth. I did not want to break our confidentiality but I thought it was necessary.

Ruth: That's okay Laura. I am not upset with you. I wanted to tell you that my granddaughter and I have come to an understanding. Although she feels the same in her beliefs, she has respected mine.

Laura: I am happy to hear that Ruth. Tammy loves you and I know her intentions were only the best.

I reached over to take Ruth's hand in mine. What a remarkable woman with an interesting past. I knew that this may be the last time I would see Ruth so I savored this moment. Soon I noticed that Ruth had fallen asleep. She looked at peace. As I entered the dining room to rejoin the others I saw that William had finished his plate. I removed his plate from the table and headed back to the kitchen. The rest of the day was spent balancing William's normal daily routine with the presence of the family.

Later that evening, I received a call from Tammy telling me that Ruth had passed. She asked if I could come in a little early the next morning to help with her father as she had arrangements to attend to. William was silent that next day and for several days that followed his mother's passing. I continued to work with William for the next couple of months until Tammy decided it was best to sell the house and move her father to a care facility.

I will always remember Ruth and her son William and the insight that I had gained from the experience. Using proper judgment when intervening in family situations requires weighing the benefits and consequences of your actions. You can not allow your emotions to lead your way. It's best to use your head first and your heart second. In this case, I feel that I had made the right decision.

True Calling
Laura Marie Patterson

Chapter 5   William – Building Trust

Related Resources

Appendix A: Building Trusting Relationships   158

Appendix F: Working with Family Members   182

Appendix E: Exercise and Social Activities   176

Related Chapters

Chapter 4: Kathy - A Family in Turmoil   40

Chapter 6: Francis - Finding Closure   102

Chapter 8: Maxine - Coping with Loss   138

Chapter 9: Dave - A Family Caregiver's Prospective 146

Chapter 6
Francis – Finding Closure

Chapter 6

Francis – Finding Closure

*W*hen I first met Francis she was in a convalescent hospital where she was recovering from hip replacement surgery. I was referred to this case by a small placement agency that I had registered with a few weeks prior. I was advised that this client was 84 year old widow that lived alone in an isolated rural home. The social worker that was assigned to her case recommended Francis have a caregiver available to her at all times if she was to return to her home.

Francis was a small petite woman but with strong features. Her hair was a silver shade of gray that was braided and neatly twisted in a bun that was pinned to the top of her head. As I approached her bed her eyes immediately looked directly into mine as to gain some insight to my intentions.

"Good Morning Francis my name is Laura. I am here to discuss the possibility of assisting you in your home once your released."

Francis: I really don't need any help. I just want to get back to my home!

Laura: That is understandable Francis. However, your doctor and nurses feel that you will need assistance in order to return to your home.

I could see the frustration building in her face as I continued to explain that this is requirement for her own safety. I also explained that my role is to prepare her meals, assist with her bathing and grooming needs and to provide transportation to her appointments.

Francis: I can see that you are a kind, responsible person, so if this is what it takes to go home and leave this God forsaken place then okay, I will accept your help.

Laura: Great! I will contact your social worker to make the necessary arrangements for your release home. In the meantime, here is my card with my phone number. Should you have any questions or concerns, please call me. I look forward to assisting and spending time with you.

Francis smiled just before I turned to walk away. It is so difficult to be separated from your home and to find yourself in unfamiliar surroundings. Recovery from any illness or surgery requires both physical and emotional healing. For an independent woman such as Francis it will be a big adjustment for her to accept my help.

I was contacted a couple days later to meet with the social worker at Francis's home. She lived in fairly large house up in the hills across from a reservoir. As I pulled up to the house I first noticed all the overgrown grass and weeds. It was obvious that the yard had not been kept up for some time. I could see a car parked halfway up the driveway that must belong to the social worker. I parked behind her car and started up the walkway towards the house.

True Calling

Laura Marie Patterson

I noticed the front door was open so I stepped in. What I saw next was shocking and a bit unsettling. There were boxes and piles of stuff stacked as high as the ceiling! Spider webs were draped from one corner of the room to the next. The smell in the room was damp and musky.

"Hello, it's Laura. Anybody here?"

I could her a voice from the back of the house call back..

"Yes, Laura. I am back here. I will be right with you"

I could hear the rustling as she made her way through the debris and towards the door where I was waiting.

"Hello, Laura. I am Linda Graves. Looks like we have a serious situation here."

Laura: Yes, unbelievable! How long has Francis been away from her home?

Linda: About 6 months.

Laura: Wow! So this is the way she lived prior to breaking her hip?

Linda: Apparently so. I can not permit her to return to a home in this condition.

Laura: That is understandable. So what do you suggest?

Linda: Well.. Either her home is cleared out, cleaned and made safe, or she will be forced to move into a long term care facility.

Laura: I see. It will take some work to accomplish the cleanup of her home. We will need her permission to do so, correct?

Linda: Yes. I will need to speak with her.

Laura: Okay. So it looks like it will be at least a couple of weeks before she can return home and only if she agrees to the cleanup.

Linda: I will give you a call and keep you up to date. Here is my card.

Laura: Thank you Linda, I look forward to hearing from you soon.

Linda locked the door behind us as we both walked out to our cars.

Laura: How could someone live like that?

Linda: It's called hoarding disorder. I have seen it a few times especially with those that live alone.

Laura: So they just can't throw anything away?

Linda: Well it's a bit more complicated than that.

Laura: This may be difficult for Francis to come to terms with. I hope it can be resolved in her best interest. Take care Linda.

True Calling
Laura Marie Patterson

Linda: Thanks for coming Laura and I will be in touch soon.

As I drove home I could not help but wonder what would lead a person to hoard? I have heard the term used before but never understood much about the disorder. I should do a little research as to have a better insight to Francis.

In the days following my discussion with Linda about Francis and her hoarding disorder, I was able to educate myself on some intervention methods. What I discovered was that hoarding is the excessive acquisition of possessions (and failure to use or discard them), even if the items are worthless, hazardous, or unsanitary. Compulsive hoarding impairs mobility and interferes with basic activities, including cooking, cleaning, showering, and sleeping.

A person who engages in compulsive hoarding is commonly said to be a "pack rat", in reference to that animal's characteristic hoarding. It is not clear whether compulsive hoarding is an isolated disorder, or rather a symptom of another condition, such as obsessive-compulsive disorder. This condition I am sure was one of the determining reasons that Francis desired to return to her own home. She was suffering not only from home sickness, but also separation anxiety from all of her possessions. It was obvious from seeing her home that most of the debris that she had collected over the years needed to be removed before it would be safe for her to return home. The second challenge would be to limit the collection of more stuff in the future which would mean a change in her own perception.

On Monday morning, I received a call from Linda. She explained that she had several discussions with Francis on what was required before she could return home.

Although she was not happy with the removal of most of her collected stuff, she did finally agree with the requirement. A cleaning crew would be arriving the next morning to remove the trash and other discards. The home would then be cleaned and arranged as to accommodate Francis and her wheelchair. I was to meet Linda on Friday morning to assist with moving Francis back into her home.

The following Friday as I drove the steep hill towards her home, I thought of the all challenges that must be addressed if Francis was to remain in her home. The initial anxiety that she will suffer once she discovers that her belongings have been disturbed will also need to be dealt with. Although this is not the ideal start for a caregiver and client relationship, I will do my best to build her trust and confidence. The first few days at home will be an adjustment period for Francis and myself as we get to know one another. As in my other client relationships of the past, it is always best to give the client space and the opportunity to discuss their needs openly.

As I approached the driveway I could see that I was the first to arrive as I had left early. After parking the car I took a look around the outside of the house. I noticed that the yard had been cleaned up and trimmed. The walkway leading to the front door was now clear of the over growth. Linda soon arrived and I could see Francis sitting in the front seat beside her with a noticeable smile on her face. I walked around to the passenger side of the car and opened the door for Francis.

Laura: Good morning Francis, I bet it's great to be back home?

Francis: We will see once I am inside!

True Calling
Laura Marie Patterson

The look of concern was obvious as she was scanning her now neatly groomed landscape.

Laura: Hello Linda. Good to see you again. Looks like the gardeners did a great job with the yard.

Linda: Yes, it looks much better.

Francis: They have destroyed my bushes!

Both Linda and myself looked at each other but did not say a word as Francis continued..

Francis: Why would someone do this without first asking me? I took care of my own yard for over 40 years and it has never looked like this!

Linda: I am sorry Francis, but we had to get the overgrowth cleared along your front walkway for your wheelchair access. Your scrubs will grow back.

Francis did not say another word as I removed her wheelchair from the trunk of Linda's car and transferred her from the passenger seat. Linda lead the way as I wheeled Francis closely behind her. Linda struggled with several keys until she finally found the one that matched the front door lock. As the door slowly creaked open, you could see the boxes that lined both sides of the entry like the walls of a fortress.

We made our way to the back of her house by way of the dining room and then through the kitchen. We entered a rather large room that appeared to have been a converted garage. There was a full size hospital bed, along with a bedside table in the corner of the room with a stand that held the television. The walls were painted stark white with no pictures or art work displayed on them. The room appeared to be very much like a hospital room and was in a neat contrast as compared to the remainder of her home.

Laura: Francis, is this where your bedroom has always been?

Francis: No my bedroom was at the other end of the house. This was my office and sewing room. Where did my sewing machine go?

Linda: It has most likely been relocated to another room in the house.

Francis: How can I ever find anything now that it has all been moved?

Laura: Once you are settled back in your home, I will be happy to help you locate your belongings that you need and put them in better order for you.

Linda: Thank you Laura, that will be most helpful for Francis. I will leave you two alone now as I have another appointment. You have my number Laura if you need anything at all please don't hesitate to call.

Laura: I appreciate all the effort you have made to accommodate Francis returning to her home. I will keep in touch as to our progress. Thanks again.

True Calling
Laura Marie Patterson

Francis: I just hope that I don't find anything missing. I use to to know where everything was, now only God knows!

Linda: Your in good hands with Laura. I am sure she will help you. I will give you a call next week. Goodbye.

After Linda had left, there was several minutes of silence as Francis quietly sat in her wheelchair and just looked around as if she was in a strange home that was not her own. I thought it was best to give her a little time before starting a conversation.

Francis: What did they do to my home? This room was a lovely shade of rose and now it is a blinding shade of white!

Laura: Perhaps they were cleaning the walls and needed to repaint. We can hang some pictures, rearrange and add to the furnishings to make you feel more at home. It may take us a little time to get things in order, but we will work on it. Looks like they have set you up with a nice comfortable hospital bed.

Francis: I want my own bed!

Laura: The hospital bed will be better for you. There are many advantages to using a bed like this.

Francis: I did not like the one in the nursing home either. They would put the rails up at night, and I felt as if I was being locked up!

Laura: The rails are used for your safety, but I can understand how it might make you feel. They have certain rules and are required to have the rails up at night. Now that your at home, perhaps it will not be necessary. I will ask the nurse what she thinks about using the rails when she visits.

Francis: Okay, but I don't have to tell you that I am not very happy about this situation. I have been away from home and my store for almost 6 months since I fell. It's good to be back home even though does not really feel like my home any longer.

Laura: Of course it's still your home. It's just has been rearranged to accommodate your wheelchair and also for your safety. You had mentioned your store?

Francis: Yes. I have owned a fabric and notions store for over 50 years.

Laura: Don't you mean you did have a store?

Francis: No. I still have a store, and I need to check on it soon!

Laura: You mean to say that you still have a store that is full of merchandise but has been unattended for six months?

Francis: Yes, that is exactly what I am telling you! I was working in the store the afternoon that I fell. A customer called 911 and they took me by ambulance to the hospital. I was on the latter reaching for a roll of fabric when I lost my balance. It was fortunate that I was not up too high when I fell, but I did end up breaking my hip.

True Calling

Laura Marie Patterson

Laura: Wow Francis, I am so to sorry hear about that. Do you own the building where your store is located?

Francis: No, I have been renting the space ever since I first opened the store in 1952. About 10 years later I expanded taking over what use to be a hair salon next door. This allowed for the fabrics in one section and the notions next door. We just created a doorway between the two buildings. My husband was very handy and built most of the shelves and counters for the store.

Laura: How long has it been since your husband passed?

Francis: He died about 8 years ago of heart failure and I had thought about closing the store at that point, but it has been such a big part of my life and has given me something to do.

Laura: So, you have continued to pay the rent on your building all the time that you have been hospitalized and in the nursing facility?

Francis: Yes, actually my business attorney has taken care of the bills. She had suggested several times that I close the store to save the $1,500.00 in rent I pay each month, but what would I ever do with all of my inventory?

Laura: Maybe you could find another fabric store that would be willing to buy it all from you? It seems like you have lost a lot of money over the last six months since your store has been closed.

Francis: I know.. but it's not just about the money. I have lots of personal things in the store as well. I just can't let some stranger come in to my store and take what they want!

Laura: I totally understand how you feel and would feel the same way myself, but this situation really needs to be resolved soon.

Francis: Barbara my attorney is coming in a few days so we can discuss it. I know she will be suggesting the same thing again.

Laura: Well.. now that you have been released there is a an opportunity for you to go through and collect your personal items before selling off the rest of your inventory?

Francis: Yes, that is what I would like to do. Would you take me down to check on my store?

Laura: I would be happy to. but first you need to get some rest for a day or two before we take a trip out. Perhaps we will discuss this first with Barbara and she might wish to accompany us.

Francis: Okay, I am a bit tired now and would like to take a nap.

Laura: Sounds like a good idea Francis. While you are resting, I will take an inventory and make a list of food items and other things that you may need.

I have read the release notes from the nursing home and in particular her dietary restrictions. Francis was on a low sodium, low sugar diet. Looking through the kitchen pantry, I noticed stacks of can goods of just about every variety. Just looking at the labels, it was obvious that these were old cans that had been purchased some time ago.

True Calling
Laura Marie Patterson

I picked up one of the cans from the front of the shelf so that I could determine an expiration date. I was shocked as I read the date of expiration stamped on the bottom of the can. "Use before 10/87" How could this can still be on her pantry shelf for almost 20 years?

The first order of business was to remove all of the expired cans. I found large refuse can out on her back patio which I promptly filled with expired cans and other outdated food items. As I had previously read about hording, the syndrome often extends to food items. This is clearly the case were Francis is concerned. While Francis was napping, it was the perfect opportunity to clean out her kitchen pantry. I will have to handle the situation delicately with Francis as I am sure throwing out these items will cause her some anxiety. Building trust with a client early on in the relationship is important. As a caregiver I have a responsibility first to my clients health and safety. I will have to work this through with Francis as well as future related issues.

Francis: Laura! Laura! Where are you?

I could hear her call from the front room where I was moving a few boxes to better clear the foyer around the door. As I approached her room I could the rattling of the bed rails

Laura: Are you okay, Francis?

Francis: Where have you been?

Laura: While you were resting, I have been taking an inventory of pantry items we need. I was also just in the front room moving a few boxes from around the front door to give us more room for your wheelchair.

Francis: Well.. I have plenty of can goods so I should be fine for sometime. I like the fruit cocktail the best.

Laura: There were several expired cans in your pantry that I needed to throw out. We can get you some fresh food items that are more healthy for you.

Francis: No! No! No! There is nothing wrong with those cans! I just open them and see if they taste "tinny". Not all of them were bad!

Laura: Francis, I can not allow you to eat expired foods. There is no reason not to have fresh fruits and vegetables. The canned foods either contain a lot of sodium or sugar which are not allowed in your diet. Wouldn't you not prefer, nice fresh steamed vegetables?

Francis: Yes, of course I like fresh fruits and vegetables, but it is always good to have a stock of can goods in case of an emergency. You never know after an earthquake or some other disaster when the stores no longer have food on their shelves. I can always rely on my supply of can foods.

Laura: We can always stock up on some new can goods. I will pick up a few cans each time I shop. I will fill your pantry again in no time. Is there a market that you like to shop near by?

Francis: There is a market that I shop just down the street from my store. I would often stop by there in the evenings after I would close my store.

Laura: Great then! I will stop by the market and possibly drive by your store along the way. Where exactly is your store located?

True Calling
Laura Marie Patterson

Francis: It's hard to miss. You just make a right on to Main Street and my store is at the corner of Oak and Main. I would like to drive out there with you.

Laura: I will tell you what.. we will both take a ride out to your store in a few days. I would like to speak with Barbara first before we go. I also want you to be well rested before we go. For today, I need to get some food items and other supplies to get us started.

Francis: Okay sounds good to me. I really miss the old place and I am hoping that no one has broken in the store while I was away.

Laura: Has Barbara been checking on the store for you?

Francis: She may have stopped by a couple of times, but she mainly just pays the rent and takes care of the business end of things.

Later that afternoon I drove out to the market and on the way stopped by to take a look at her store. I parked my car around the back behind the store and walked around to the front of the store to take a look through the front window. As I approached the store, I noticed the display that remained in the front window. There were small American flags stuck in blocks of Styrofoam to hold them for display. Red, white and blue fabric was carefully draped over what appeared to be cardboard boxes. It was obvious that this display was intended for the 4th of July holiday. This would follow the time-line of when Francis had fallen in the store. It is now mid February and the display looks oddly out of place.

Looking through the glass door and down the darkened aisle of the store, I noticed the sturdy metal shelves with stacks of fabric reams that reached to the ceiling. Without entering the store, I could tell from peeking inside that there was a tremendous amount of stock. I could not help but wonder what will she do with all of the store's merchandise? I am sure that these are issues that Barbara will be addressing when she visits. I stood there a few minutes visualizing Francis as she worked in her store, helping customers selecting from the many patterns of fabric that she sold. Francis had invested fifty years of her life into her business. It is easy to understand the emotional attachment that she has for her store.

After leaving her store I went to the market to fill my shopping list. I purchased vegetables, fruit, along with fish and chicken. I also picked up a couple cans of low sodium beans and canned fruit without added sugar. These were purchased not as intended meal items but to place on her pantry shelves as I promised. Building trust with a client often involves the little but important things such as following through on promises. To most of us a couple cans of beans may be unimportant, but to Francis it represented security. I will build a trusting relationship with Francis one day at a time.

Upon returning from shopping, I heard rustling from the back of the house. As I entered the room, I could see Francis as she was bent over a a stack of newspapers that was piled under the card table located in the corner of her room.

Laura: What are you up to Francis?

Francis: Thank goodness they did not throw out my newspapers!

True Calling
Laura Marie Patterson

Laura: They look old and yellowed. Are they collectable or of some personal importance?

Francis: No, just never got around to clipping the recipes and comics that I wanted from them.

I reached down as picked up one of the newspapers. As I scanned the headlines I noted the date, September 14th, 1967. This newspaper was almost 40 years old!

Laura: Where do you put these clippings once they have been cut out?

Francis: I have three boxes in my closet. One for the recipes, one for the comics and the third box is for miscellaneous clippings or gardening hints. One day, I hope to go through those boxes and place them into folders, but for now I need to get these finished and stored in boxes.

Laura: I see.. your a well organized person. I stopped by your store and looked through the front window. You have an amazing selection of fabrics from what I could see. I also liked your 4th of July window display too. Very creative.

Francis: Oh my! I need to change that display!

Laura: I don't think at this point it is a priority since the store has already been closed for over six months.

Francis: Don't talk to me about priorities young lady! I have been in business at the same location for over fifty years so I know how to manage my priorities!

Laura: I am sorry Francis, I did not mean to offend you. I was only suggesting that you need to discuss this and other issues with Barbara on Friday when she visits. I am sure that she has thought about your options and will discuss them with you.

Francis: She does not run my business, I do! She is only good for making sure that my sales tax forms are filed and my bank statements are balanced. When it comes to making decisions about retail merchandising or advertising, that is my department.

Laura: Okay Francis, I understand. This is a difficult time for you as things are so unsettled. Don't worry, I know it will take a little time to sort this all out. I am sure you will get it all worked out soon.

Francis: It can't happen too soon for me!

Friday morning Barbara arrived as scheduled. Barbara was a tall well dressed woman with vibrant red hair neatly arranged about her shoulders. She carried herself in a authoritative manner and was well spoken and direct. I remained in the kitchen while their meeting took place, but was within hearing distance of their conversation. It was especially easy to over hear the parts where Francis objected to closing her store and donating the remaining merchandise to charity. It was apparent from their discussion that neither of the two were in agreement as to the future of the store.

True Calling
Laura Marie Patterson

After about an hour, Barbara left the room. As she came through the kitchen on her way to the front door, she motioned to me to follow her. I walked closely behind and soon as we were out on the front porch, Barbara turned to me with a serious look on her face.

Barbara: Laura, normally I would never discuss my client's business without their permission, however in this case I wish to make an exception. As you know, Francis has owned a fabric store for many years. Since her hospitalization it has been closed, and I had no choice in the interim but to continue to pay the store rent and related expenses.

Laura: If you don't mind my asking, how much is the rent per month?

Barbara: She has a lease with the owner of the building on a five year term. She is now in the last year of her lease and her monthly rent is 1,500.00. There is also utilities and the required insurance. This brings the monthly expenses to around 1,900.00.

Laura: So how may I help?

Barbara: I feel she needs to have an opportunity discuss the reality of the situation with a neutral party. Possibility you could suggest some of the options that I discussed with her this afternoon?

Laura: I could not hear your discussion very clearly, what might those options be?

Barbara: The most practical option would be for her to donate the merchandise which the benefactors would be responsible for the removal of the merchandise and moving out the fixtures. This way, the building could be turned back over to the owner quickly. I will still have to negotiate the termination of her lease, but I do know the owner of the building has expressed an interest in a tenant that wants to open a pizza parlor in that location.

Laura: How receptive was Francis to her suggestion?

Barbara: Not very. She feels that by donating her store merchandise she is giving away part of her life. This is a very emotional decision for her. As her caregiver your participation in discussing this option could be helpful for her to come to terms with the reality and urgency of the situation.

Laura: Okay Barbara, I will offer my support to her. She needs to deal with this unsolved issue soon as it is causing her obvious distress.

Barbara: Thank you Laura. Here is my card with my office and cellphone number. Please call if you need anything. I really appreciate your assistance.

I stood on the front porch as I watched Barbara get into her Mercedes coupe and back out of the long driveway. What could I say to convince Francis to move forward with closing a very long and important chapter in her life? I do know one thing for sure, Francis is very strong willed and not easily swayed.

True Calling
Laura Marie Patterson

The next morning after breakfast, Francis and I took a little stroll out to her front porch and around the back of the house to the garden that is now dormant from the winter cold. Although brisk, the sun felt warm on our faces and close by I found an old plastic lawn chair that I dusted off, and pulled the chair next to Francis as she sat in her wheelchair.

Laura: It's beautiful out this morning Francis. You have so many birds in the yard, how wonderful!

Francis: Yes, you should see them in the spring. I am usually out here most mornings with bread crumbs feeding them. I have many animals that visit here that I call my pets, all but the skunks of course!

We both laughed and talked about how her and her husband bought the home back in the 1950's and all the work it took to clear the "back 5", meaning the five acres behind their home. "We would work most weekends and holidays back here. It was a working vacation as we would call it.", said Francis as she gazed passed the rickety fence that separated the yard grass from the rustic area lined with tall trees.

Laura: This is quite a large home and yard to maintain on your own. Between running your store and your home's upkeep, you certainly have your hands full. Now that your health has changed and your a bit older, you need to make some changes in your lifestyle and physical exertion.

Francis: Yes, I know that breaking my hip is forcing me to slow down a bit from my previous pace, but it will not stop me in my tracks! I have a gardener for the yard, a housekeeper that comes once a week to help with the house and a high school girl that would help out at the store in the afternoons and Saturdays.

Laura: Sound like you had things well worked out for yourself. Have you thought about your plans for the future?

Francis: As you may have heard, I had a heated discussion with Barbara on this subject. I refuse to give away all that I have worked so hard for the last 50 years. I was planning on retiring the store in a couple years, that is why I have not ordered stock in the last few years. I was planning on selling the existing merchandise until most of it was gone. Then I would finally close the store and that chapter of my life.

Laura: Yes Francis and a long chapter it has been. I can understand your feeling about an abrupt closure of your store and the donation of your merchandise. Maybe there is another alternative to Barbara's suggestion?

Francis: Like what?

Laura: Have you thought about selling the store?

Francis: I did have one lady that was interested in buying the place, but at the time I did not seriously entertain the thought.

Laura: How long ago was that?

True Calling
Laura Marie Patterson

Francis: It has been several years ago. I really don't want to hand the store over to someone that would possibly destroy the great reputation that has taken me fifty years to build. I would rather just close the store all together than to allow that to happen.

Laura: Okay, here's an idea. Why not hire a manager and a couple of girls to reopen the store and sell the remaining stock?

Francis: I don't think I could find someone that I could trust and that would not rob me blind!

Laura: I can understand your trust issues, but what if you were still able to play an active roll in the management of the store?

Francis: So what are you suggesting then?

Laura: Why don't you and I open the store back up on a part-time basis and see what we can do? Maybe we could hire someone to help us out?

Francis: I don't know.. I will have to think about this awhile.

Laura: Okay, I will tell you what. Why don't we go out to the store tomorrow? I know you are wanting to check on the store and I would love to see the inside from beyond the windows.

A big smile came upon her face and she agreed that she has been anxious to check on the condition of her store.

The rest of the day was filled with stories of the customers that frequented her store over the years. As she would tell these stories you could see the pride on her face. Francis needed closure and it was obvious from her reaction that it would not be accomplished by abruptly closing her store and donating her merchandise.

The next morning after breakfast we set out to visit the store. As we pulled around the back of the building to park the car, you could see a large smile begin to grow on her face. I had placed the wheelchair in the trunk and her walker folded in the backseat of my car.

Francis: You will have to unlock the backdoor from inside the store. Here are the keys to the store. The lights are turned on from the panel behind the door in the office. Walk straight back then the door is on the right.

Laura: Okay, wait here in the car and I will come through the store and unlock the back door for us.

As I took the short walk around the building, my thoughts reflected back to many stories that Francis had told me about the store. This will be a difficult transition for her. I fumbled with the many keys on the ring until I found the right key that fit the front door. As I walked to the back of the store towards the office, I again noticed that many rolls of fabric that lined the shelves, were mostly covered with a thin layer of dust.

I opened the door to the office to find an old oak desk with a swivel chair. On the desk was an adding machine, the kind with the lever that you pull for the results. Across from the desk was a folding card table with several plastic small drawer organizers filled with what appeared to be buttons of every style and color.

True Calling
Laura Marie Patterson

As I turned around, I saw the light panel just to the right of the door as Francis described. I turned each switch on one at a time until the store was brightly lit. I walked through the stockroom to the back of the store. I was amazed at the additional rolls of fabric and the stacks of boxes that were stored. The store was a reflection of her home. Packed to the ceiling and with no unused space.

I struggled with opening the back door as the hinges seemed rusted as the door slowly creaked open.

I walked around to the back of my car and pulled the wheelchair from the trunk. Francis was visibly anxious as I carefully assisted her to the wheelchair and wheeled her into the store.

Francis: Oh my! The store is so dingy!

Laura: Yes.. after 6 months of no upkeep, things do tend to get a bit dusty. We can hire a few people and have this place in tip top shape in no time.

Francis: I have not decided to sell the store so I don't see the point?

Laura: Remember the idea I suggested? Why don't we re-open the store a couple days a week and see what we can do? You can always make the decision to sell later but for now an open store would sell much easier than a dirty closed one. What do you think?

Francis: Your really willing to do this with me?

Laura: Sure, why not? It sure beats cutting out newspaper clippings!

126

In the course of the following week we were able to hire two neighbor high school girls to help us clean and straighten the store. By the end of the week the store was ready for the grand re-opening. I thought of a new marketing strategy that would make the out dated fabrics and old store merchandise more appealing. We would rename the store from "Main Street Fabrics & Notions" to "Vintage Fancy Fabrics & Buttons". We placed an ad in the local paper announcing the event and the newspaper was interested in writing an article on Francis and her fifty years at the same location. As it turned out, the store had a real following as it had been a town fixture for so many years. The article talked about the many generations of mothers, daughters and housewives that had depended on Francis and her store to supply their sewing needs.

Business was swift as many would visit the store to just say hello to Francis and leave with an arm load of goods. Originally we planned on reopening the store on Mondays, Wednesdays and Friday, but soon expanded our hours to include Saturdays as well. In order to give Francis the rest she needed, we hired Toni, a high school girl to help us out on Saturdays. Francis would sit in her wheelchair working the cash register as I would help the customers and cut the fabric. I was never much of a seamstress, but over time I gained a real knowledge of notions and fabrics.

The store remained open for over a year and half until Francis was unfortunately diagnosed with cancer. By that time we were able to sell the majority of the store's merchandise. Although the store never really turned much of a profit, we were able to at least break even with the store rent and expenses. Most importantly, It was an enjoyable experience for the both of us while giving Francis much needed closure.

True Calling
Laura Marie Patterson

Shortly after her diagnosis, the cancer really started to progress so it was necessary to move her to a skilled nursing facility where she would receive the hospice care as needed. I continued working with Francis keeping an eye on her home and coordinating the closing of her store. We initially moved the remaining store merchandise to storage until it was eventually donated to a charity.

Francis passed away one rainy October day ending the life of an extraordinary strong willed and independent woman. She had no immediate family as she never had children. A distant relative from out of state was her benefactor and attended her funeral service along with a few close neighbors and friends. I will never forget the busy days spent at the store nor the off beat jokes and laughter that we both often shared. Our lives are filled with challenges and accomplishments. As we reach the end of our lives, we have these to reflect upon and finding closure is equally as important.

True Calling
Laura Marie Patterson

Chapter 6 Francis – Finding Closure

Related Resources

Appendix A: Building Trusting Relationships   158

Appendix B: Safety in the Home and Hidden Dangers 162

Appendix C: Nutrition and Food Preparation   166

Appendix E: Exercise and Social Activities   176

Related Chapters

Chapter 5: William - Building Trust   70

Chapter 7: Sam - His Strong Will to Live   132

This page was left blank intentionally.

Chapter 7
Sam – His Strong Will To Live

Chapter 7

Sam – His Strong Will To Live

I began caring privately for a gentleman that was diagnosed with a rare condition called Shy Drager's Syndrome. This neurological disorder is similar to Parkinson's Disease but attacks mainly the central and autonomic nervous systems which causes incontinence, constipation and a sudden drop in blood pressure when standing. When I was contacted for this case I was told that the client was currently under the care of Hospice and that his prognosis for longevity may be just a few weeks. I was to watch over him and report any serious changes in his condition. He was under nourished and suffered from numerous pressure sores as a result of being bed confined. Even though Sam was in such a dire condition, he had a smile and spirit about him that could light up the room. He just was not ready to give in to his illness as he still had a strong will to live.

Sam was diagnosed with Shy Drager's Syndrome approximately 8 years before. The life expectancy of this disease is between 7-8 years, so his doctors had little hope for Sam's improved condition.

Sam and I talked for hours about his life and his strong desire to survive. At the time at the the time I began caregiving for Sam, he was 83 and married 50 + years to a wonderful woman that had been his caregiver prior to my arrival. The years of stress and uncertainty had taken it's toll on her and she just did not have the emotional or physical ability to continue with his care. Unfortunately, this also lead to Sam's rapid decline as well.

I promised Sam I would do all I could to help him be comfortable and have the best quality of life possible. I also told him that we need to work together to achieve these goals. We were able to establish a bond and trust that enabled a slow but steady improvement in Sam's condition. Within a few weeks he had gained 10 pounds and was sitting up and was able to move in bed which allowed for the treatment and healing of his pressure sores. Within 2 months he was removed from Hospice and placed in Palliative Care.

Another on-going issue for Sam was his Dementia which was accompanied by acute short term memory loss. Although, he would remember my face, he could not remember my name. On the weekends when his grandchildren would visit, he would mention their visitation but could not associate who they really were.

He would talk of how he and his wife had met. An elaborate tale of meeting her on a street corner when he was stationed in Hawaii. He told me that he would see her around town several times before he actually mustered up the courage to ask her on a date. According to Sam, Carmen was many years his junior and this was part of his reluctance in getting involved with a girl her age. Later, when speaking with Carmen, I recounted Sam's story. She told me that they had met before he was stationed in Hawaii and that she had never lived there. She told me that they had met at a office where she had worked before Sam's enlistment in the Navy.

Often times dementia patients become confused and makeup stories to fill in missing memories. Because of their confusion their fantasized stories becomes their own reality. Sam believed these stories as fact and surprisingly stayed true to the details each time he would repeat the story.

True Calling
Laura Marie Patterson

After learning the truth, I never confronted Sam by correcting his facts. An individual with dementia could see this as a confrontation and a negative action thus damaging the delicate balance of trust between his or her caregiver.

There are many activities that can be shared that are very beneficial to short term memory loss. Puzzles are a great way to exercise the mind by challenging reason. Avoid large picture puzzles with many pieces in favor of simple picture puzzles with fewer pieces. It is important to give encouragement and a feeling of accomplishment as well. I purchased a couple of puzzles that were designed for young children. I was able to find puzzles with pictures of airplanes, cars and wild animals. I would give Sam one puzzle at a time and would rotate them every couple of days. At first Sam would not remember the puzzle that he had previously put together, but before long he would recognize the pictures. He would challenge himself by how fast he could put the puzzle together. We started with 25 piece puzzles and soon graduated to more complicated 100 piece puzzles.

Sam was a talented carpenter and handyman and would take pride in his tools that he still maintained hanging above his work bench in the garage. On several occasions, he would ask to go into the garage where he would explain what each of the tools were used for. I was amazed at the progress that was made with his memory and soon he was calling me by my first name.

Each morning Sam and I would go out to the back patio and feed the birds. Sam loved to feel the warm morning sunshine on his face. We also went for short walks to the front yard and then around the side of the house to the backyard.

Sam

His Strong Will To Live

Although Sam was confined to his wheelchair for the most part, he could stand and walk for short distances with the assistance of his walker. This exercise was important to keep his leg muscles from weaking and to aid in his blood circulation.

He would tell me of his adventures in World War II and how he had piloted P-51 aircraft. For his birthday that first year, I bought him a model airplane that we had built together and later hung above his bed. He was very proud of the completed model and had much pride in showing it off to his grand children when they visited.

As the months went by Sam's condition had continued to improve which baffled his nurses and physicians. I started bringing my guitar with me almost daily, since Sam himself had played the violin when he was younger and enjoyed music so much. I brought a tambourine and maracas which Sam would use to accompany my guitar playing. Pretty soon Sam and I had several songs that we had practiced and would perform them for family and friends.

The miracle of Sam's recovery and longevity can only be contributed to his strong will to live combined with an overall better quality of life.

Sam did pass of congestive heart failure 2 1/2 years later. However, the time that Sam and I had shared together and his infectious smile will remain in my heart forever.

True Calling
Laura Marie Patterson

Chapter 7 Sam – His Strong Will to Live

Related Resources

Appendix A: Building Trusting Relationships   158

Appendix C: Nutrition and Food Preparation   166

Appendix D: Dementia and Memory Loss   170

Appendix E: Exercise and Social Activities   176

Appendix F: Working with Family Members   182

Related Chapters

Chapter 2: Jimmy and Sabrina - Their Commitment   14

Chapter 5: William - Building Trust   70

Chapter 6: Francis - Finding Closure   102

Chapter 8
Maxine – Coping With Loss

Chapter 8

Maxine – Coping With Loss

*W*hen I first started working with Maxine, the days were filled with stories of how she had met her husband Jack, their trip around the world, and his accomplishments with the humanities department at San José State University.

(Maxine had just lost her husband of 52 years, just four months prior. Still fresh in her mind, I could see the difficulty she was having in dealing with her loss.)

A big part of her husband's life outside of their marriage, was his involvement with the formation of the humanities department. My interest was sparked in doing some research on my own, so I visited the San José State University's website where I found no information available as to the history of the humanities program or it's founders.

When I told Maxine about the absence of any historical reference, she was disappointed that Jack's contribution to such an important program at San Jose State could be lost for the future generations of students. I decided to contact San José State to ask if there were any plans to update the humanities section on their website with some historical background information. I was contacted by the secretary for the Dean of Humanities and was told that the idea will be discussed.

As caregivers we must be able to put ourselves in the clients place as to have a better understanding and empathy to what he or she is feeling emotionally. Most of us would have a very difficult time even imagining what it would be like to have lost our mate of over 50 years. Depending on how soon the loss has occurred and if there is strong support of family and friends, it can make a real difference in the initial grieving period. Since Maxine had lived in the same home for most of her marriage, she had a strong network of neighborhood friends that were very helpful in the initial days and weeks following Jacks passing.

Having been placed with a client that has suffered this kind of personal loss, it is important that I continue to support and nurture Maxine's recovery from her grief. One of the ways I helped Maxine was to have conversations about her life before she had met her husband Jack. Talking about her life and self accomplishments before her marriage is a way for her to visualize that life is possible after losing her husband.

Planning social activities such as visiting friends and shopping trips are both a great distraction from her loss and reinforces her ability to have an independent life of her own. We would always plan on setting Fridays aside to have a fun day out and away from the house.

Since the death of her husband occurred 2 days before what would have been his 92nd birthday, once a month around the 25th we would visit his grave site to bring flowers and to pay tribute to his memory. Afterwords we try to couple this activity with something enjoyable like having lunch out or shopping.

True Calling
Laura Marie Patterson

On the 23rd of March which also marked the one year anniversary of his death, we planned a small picnic at the memorial park where he was buried. I brought my guitar and played a classical piece since Jack was also an accomplished musician and had played in the local symphony for many years. This was a fitting addition to our "celebration of life" in his honor and added enjoyment to an otherwise somber occasion.

A few months later, we were contacted by San José State, to discuss the idea further with Maxine. They were also interested in any information that she could share with them about Jack's early involvement with the humanities department since all of the original professors have since passed.

Maxine was delighted at the prospect of Jack being recognized for all his professional accomplishments. Together we looked through boxes of memorabilia in an effort to collect as much information as we could. We also found newspaper articles and pictures in a scrapbook that would be very helpful in documenting the history of the humanities honors program. I made copies of these clippings and photos that went back as far as 1954. I then organized the material in a folder to present to the historical committee.

Jack's associate in the humanities pilot program was Clint Williams. Unfortunately, Professor Williams and his wife had passed away a few years prior, so any additional information about the program would be difficult to obtain.

Maxine did mention that the Williams had a son that was also a college professor at another university. With this knowledge I was able to use the Internet to track the William's son down in Florida where he was now retired and living on his boat. I sent him an email explaining of our intentions and he was very helpful in verifying some additional information about both his father and Jacks involvement with the creation of the humanities honors program.

A meeting was arranged at Maxine's home with San Jose State a few weeks later. The current Dean of Humanities was present along with some administrators involved with the historical project. We had a fascinating discussion about the history of San José State University and the importance of the humanity honors program. It was also decided that in addition to the website update, a plaque naming the founders of the humanities honors program and their pictures should be displayed honoring these Professors. As you can only imagine Maxine was overjoyed with the prospect of having Jack and the other professors honored permanently on a plaque and displayed on campus at San Jose State University.

In the weeks that followed, additional discussions took place both by email and by phone. One day, Maxine and I were discussing the wives of the professors and the important role that they played in supporting their husbands during that challenging period of developing the humanities honors program. In our discussion, Maxine mentioned that the wives should also be honored for their part as well.

True Calling

Laura Marie Patterson

We took a sheet of paper and made a drawing of what it would look like to have the professors photos above and just below another photo of each of "The Women Behind The Men". We both laughed about the actual possibility, but little did I know at the time that Maxine was taking that idea very seriously and would later mention this to the Dean of the Humanities at a social dinner.

It has now been almost a year since our idea was first proposed to San José State University and soon it will become a reality. There will be a series of four portraits. The two founding professors, Clint Williams and Jack Fink, followed by the two professors that followed them in the program will be displayed on the plaque. Below each professor's photo will be a portrait of their wife.

The plaque will have the following inscription:

"Founded in 1954, the Humanities Honors program remains one of the most innovative and successful educational endeavors in the history of San José State University. From the beginning, Humanities Honors courses were guided by a team of four outstanding instructors who brought a rich, interdisciplinary approach to General Education and humanistic consciousness. This plaque commemorates the pioneering team of Humanities Honors professors: O.C. "Clint" Williams, Jack E. Fink, Richard Tansey and Rex Burbank and their greatly supportive wives: Elisabeth "Betsy" Willaims, Maxine Hunt Fink, Luraine Tansey and Nancy Burbank."

Maxine

I am so happy that Jack and the other three professors will finally be recognized for their historic contribution to San Jose State University's history.

Elisabeth Kübler-Ross, M.D. described in her 1969 book (On death and dying), "denial, anger, bargaining, depression and acceptance, are the five stages of grief." In Maxine's case, I have witnessed her transcend through four of those five stages. There is no definite time-line in dealing with grief and loss. Only as we transcend through each of the stages, can we start to experience acceptance.

As of this writing I am still working with Maxine as we have developed a very close relationship over the last year and half. We have achieved goals, endured the sadness and have shared the laughter. After all, caregiving is so much more than providing daily care. It's sharing in experiences and improving the client's quality of life.

True Calling
Laura Marie Patterson

Chapter 8 Maxine - Coping With Loss

Related Resources

Appendix A: Building Trusting Relationships   158

Appendix E: Exercise and Social Activities   176

Appendix G: Supporting Loss and Grief   186

Appendix H: Caring for the Caregiver   194

Related Chapters

Chapter 5: William - Building Trust   70

Chapter 6: Francis - Finding Closure   102

Chapter 9
Dave – A Family Caregiver's Perspective

True Calling

Laura Marie Patterson

The following chapter was written by a husband that has been caring for his wife for several years. I met David through an online family caregiving support forum and I was moved by his unconditional love and dedication to his wife. I asked David if he would be willing to share his perspective through a family caregiver's point of view, and he graciously accepted.

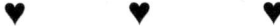

♥　　♥　　♥

"Your wife has had a stroke." That call from the ER doctor many years ago started my caregiving journey. My name is Dave and I care for my wife Pat. My wife is not a client, she is the love of my life.

My first reaction was anger. My wife actually had the stroke on Friday and the ER Doctor had misdiagnosed her. So we went home and toughed out the weekend. I was scheduled for a business trip the next week and she insisted that I go. Monday night some friends came over and seeing her condition immediately took her back to the hospital. This time she was accurately diagnosed but I was a couple hundred of miles away. Amazingly she recovered from that stroke with only a little weakness. But her health continued to decline and soon she developed Peripheral Artery Disease, foot ulcers and Congestive Heart Failure among other things mostly as a result of diabetes. Today she is in a wheelchair, cannot drive and must have assistance to leave the house.

Being a family caregiver is different from that of a paid caregiver. There are no days off. My days start early and end late. On weekdays we awaken at 6:00 AM. First thing is to make sure my wife is awake and can safely get out of bed.

My wife is at a high risk of falling. Tangled blankets can and have caused her to fall. Then it's off to the bathroom to do my morning rituals while she is getting ready in the bedroom. She has a bedside commode for safety and to prevent accidents. After finishing up in the bathroom I return and help her dress as I'm getting dressed. Then we get ready to go to her hyperbolic treatment. We go out to our minivan and after making sure she transfers safely from her wheelchair to the van we then load the wheelchair and drive to the treatment center. At the treatment center I help her transfer and get ready for her treatment. Then she starts hyperbolic treatment and I go to work. When my wife gets home she sends me an instant message that she is back safely. We use instant messaging to communicate, as it is less disruptive to my workday. During the day we can message back and forth in case of troubles. We also have a retired older gentleman who lives with us who watches my wife during the day.

After work I have to do shopping, as I am the only one who can drive. If my wife is feeling well she may go along, but most times she does not. Then it's home for supper sometimes it's ready and sometimes I have to cook. The evening is spent doing things around the house and helping my wife. This may include housework, handyman work, getting her dressed, personal things and getting pills ready. If her foot hurts I may have to change bandages or put lotion on her to protect her skin. We have been fighting a loosing battle to keep her business going and some nights I work on that as well.

On a good day I get to watch TV for an hour or so. On a bad day I just go to bed and sleep. It's not the physical challenges but the unrelenting nature of the work that is my biggest challenge.

True Calling
Laura Marie Patterson

We are luckier than most in that we have a lot of friends who come over to visit and help with things. This is a huge thing for a caregiver and our friends are a tremendous help. They mostly help with taking my wife shopping and picking up things for her. Indeed sometimes I can get a friend that will stay with her so I can do things. Most importantly our friends provide her with the social contact she needs to keep her health and spirits up. Lastly, they pray for us. As Christians this means a lot to us.

Weekends are similar but I do sleep in till 7am. Then it's up and get dressed for the home health nurse. Saturday is the day I usually do larger projects around the house and then get ready for church it is also my resting day. Sunday is church and though my duties there have been cut so that I can care for my wife, it's still a busy day that is devoted to serving God.

As a family caregiver there are a lot of differences from coming and doing it as a job. Not better or worse, just different. We don't get time off. Family caregivers are on duty 24/7 and it's unrelenting. Mornings and evenings my wife out of necessity comes first, then my priorities are second. Trying to say "This is my time" can have very bad consequences, especially if she is having difficulty with a transfer she can fall and injure herself. It is all but impossible to sit down and concentrate on a long task as there are calls to help my wife. Getting her into bed or out of bed, checking on pills, talking to the doctor or home health nurse, helping her get ready or help with a transfer that is not working. These are in addition to normal household chores. I use the DVR to record shows, it allows me to stop them when a call for help comes. Being on constant call is not too bad for a short time, but when it goes on and on for months and years without let-up, it never allows you to have any time for yourself.

Professional caregivers often have limited responsibility and a specific area of care. Family caregivers have no such limitations and are doing far more complex medical things than ever before. Medical care providers are very conscious of costs these days and often to reduce them will push more and more duties on to patients and their families as represent to them, "free labor". As part of the daily care for my wife I have to change dressings on her foot. This is not a simple manner of swapping a bandage strip. Her foot dressing takes a full roll of gauze and at the end looks like a sock made of gauze. This is to cover multiple wounds. Also to prevent infection, you must scrub and wear gloves during the procedure. In addition, wounds must be cleaned and ointments must be applied in a certain way to assist in healing. It takes 15-30 minutes to change a dressing on her foot. In addition you must keep an eye out for signs of infection or loss of circulation. You must advise the medical people if you find anything unusual.

Medications are another difficult area we have pills, patches, inhalers and shots that all must be administered and monitored. I'm just using what I do as an example, many family caregivers are doing jobs that in the past would have been provided by nurses and other trained professionals.

Family caregivers pay a financial price as well. Most family caregivers generally are middle class and are not rich. Although we may have a good job, we will pay a price financially for having a chronically ill loved one. Most chronically ill people cannot hold a job, so this limits them usually to Social Security Disability. The caregiver will loose out on income in their job as well. We can't take overtime if it suddenly comes available because we have to be home for our loved ones.

True Calling
Laura Marie Patterson

Travel for any reason is also difficult. In days past, I traveled throughout North America and sometimes other places this allowed me to make extra money. Today trying to get away for an overnight trip requires a lot of arrangements. Even worse you will be spending more on your reduced income. My wife's illness requires a copay for prescriptions, van transport for my wife when I am working and no reimbursement for some medical supplies. Total costs are from $300 to $400 a month. One surprising area is vehicle costs. To transport my wife we must take a minivan, some have larger vans as well. I was lucky in that I was able to adapt our van myself to transport my wife. Even without the expense of modifications we still pay extra for fuel every week because we cannot use a smaller and more fuel efficient car. We also have the issue of assets. Most state programs are dependent on your income and assets. If you have a good job or assets you will not qualify for many government programs.

A well meaning person asked why I don't put my wife in a nursing home. I gently explained that even if we agreed on one, under Medicaid rules that most of my 401k would be taken to pay for her nursing home care before Medicaid would kick in. The costs given are just an example, since my finances are better than many family caregivers. Many family caregivers struggle at or below the poverty line. But no matter what your income, finances are always an area of stress for family caregivers.

Emotions are also a huge issue. For family caregivers there are no patients or clients. There are wives and husbands, mothers and fathers, sons and daughters, brothers and sisters, grandfathers and grandmothers. The point is that they are people who we have a pre-existing emotional relationship with.

There are several issues this causes. There is the pain of seeing a loved one suffer. This means watching someone who you care for in pain. Watching them loose physical and or mental abilities. This is painful to watch as nobody wants to see a loved one slowly lose functions and the personality that we have loved so much. My wife has lost much of her ability to function in the past, as she often drove especially on long trips. We both preferred it that way. She used to be very strong and able to move things around the house with little or no help. Both of those things are now distant memories. She is unlikely to completely recover, so like many caregivers we are fighting a losing battle.

Our goal is to keep fighting for as long as we can. The ones we care for are often irritable. Pain and illness are not pleasant things to go through. People understandably become irritable and angry. Though we understand it with our heads, it takes it's toll on our hearts over the months and years. The mental component of many illnesses can take its toll on us as well. During a recent hospitalization an infection rendered my wife very confused and out of touch with reality. The hospital called to ask me to come over and calm her down. I very quickly left work and to talk to my wife. She had lost all touch with reality and was dangerous to herself and everybody around her. She was facing off the whole staff including security. She was angry and confused and was trying to leave the hospital. Finally we got a major tranquilizer that calmed her down so we could treat her. When you see that happen to someone you love it's not the kind of thing you forget easily. That was a good hospital. At bad hospitals, you may deal with staff that may mistreat your loved one.

True Calling
Laura Marie Patterson

Those same people may regard you as nothing more than an annoying pest. At one hospital, I came in and found my wife laying in her own waste! I went to the staff very upset to get her cleaned up. Needless to say, we did not go back to that hospital anymore.

All of this would take a toll on an ideal relationship. Many times relationships are far from ideal. You have all the baggage from previous problems compounded by the stress of caregiving. We struggle with that and the upending of relationships and the blurring of lines. We used to have a traditional marriage. I went to work and she took care of things around the house and we liked it that way. Today our relationship is more of caregiving for my wife as bravely she does all she can do, but this is very limited compared to the past. Ultimately, all of these relationships become more parental in nature. For parents and children it is even worse as the relationship is upended with the children becoming parents. Then there is guilt. There is usually no good reason for it, but we feel guilty anyway. Guilty in why didn't it happen to us? Guilt in, why can't we do more? Guilt in why we can't have unending patience? Guilt because we have to work, and guilt based on our past relationships. Guilt is our daily companion. Most family caregivers bear a heavy and hidden emotional load. Family caregivers are in it for the long haul. Our caregiving assignment ends usually with the death of our loved one. Our assignments are not for weeks and months, but for years and decades. At the end we don't get a new assignment, we get the stages of grief while trying to put our own shattered lives back together.

So how do you deal with a family caregiver? It's easy, it takes very little to make a caregivers day. Realize that we are busy with our loved ones and most of the time our goal is to make it through the day. We don't have time for a lot of other things. Be understanding, we appreciate it. But don't say you understand how we feel unless you have actually done family caregiving. Instead say, "I'm here for you." Go and visit them, as long term illness and caregiving tend to isolate people. We would like to visit you as well, but for us visits are difficult. We most often have specialized equipment to deal with the medical needs of our loved ones in our own homes. Your home most likely does not have that equipment, meaning that we must not only transport our loved ones but the equipment that we need. Simple access can be a problem. We have adapted our homes to be wheelchair friendly, most houses are not wheelchair friendly. This makes it a lot harder for us to leave and visit. In addition, our loved ones can get very tired and weak quickly without warning. It's a lot easier on us to just put them in their own bed. Offering to help with shopping is always welcome either by taking people shopping or by picking something up. If appropriate, you could also try other chores as well such as bathing or personal care. Just be sure you are capable of doing the task. But the most important thing is to visit. A regular friendly visit does a home-bound person a world of good.

Professional and family caregivers have a complex relationship. Good professional caregivers are gems. But like gems they are rare. We now have some excellent caregivers for my wife and working as a team. She is getting the best of care possible, but it is was a struggle to get to this point and it remains a struggle to keep things in place. If you are a professional don't necessarily expect a warm welcome.

True Calling
Laura Marie Patterson

We have had some excellent caregivers for my wife, but we have also had some very bad ones. When you first arrive I'm cool but watchful looking for the things that make an excellent caregiver. Here's what I'm looking for; Are you reliable? Can I count on you arriving when you say you will? That does not always mean a set time, we are willing to be flexible. Are you doing appropriate and safe work? You need to work safely with my wife, while dropping her during a transfer will likely result in your not being invited back. Likewise you do not need to go through all her dresser drawers. Supplies are kept in a known location we will tell you where they are.

On the subject of supplies are you watching the levels? We do keep some backups, but understand these come out of our own money. Most of the time when we buy supplies we are not reimbursed for them. Medications are important as well. The pharmacy will do an emergency refill if needed but we try not to make every refill an emergency. Are you communicating with me? As a family caregiver one of my important jobs is to facilitate communication among our team. I would appreciate your cell number and of course you can have mine. The reason is that when my wife is in the hospital I will send a daily text message that will advise you of what is happening and when to expect her home, and this allows you to set your schedule. Also if you see something, say something. Medical problems often start very small and can be easily treated if we know about them. Ignoring small symptoms results in hospitalization or worst.

One time I called the home health nurse and told her my wife was in the hospital for pneumonia. Her response was, "I'm not surprised I heard her lungs filling up." After asking why in heaven's name she didn't bother to tell anyone, we got a new agency. Communication is very important it can prevent hospitalization and make home health a better and cheaper option.

Lastly remember that this is a team effort. Make the effort to find where you fit in and be flexible. Any professional caregiver that is reliable and keeps up with supplies, communicates well, and works as a team, is not only welcome in this house but also respected.

I've learned many things over the years of caregiving. While finishing this chapter, my wife after many years had stroke symptoms. But only some symptoms. She was missing many of the "classic" symptoms. We watched them and finally called the ambulance. The paramedics evaluated her and were not sure that she was having a stroke and asked if we wanted her taken to the hospital. I told them it was a judgment call, but yes. After she was checked out, the diagnoses came back a very minor stroke. Thankfully it did not affect her very much. There were many differences about this hospital stay than the first one. The knowledge that we now have is beneficial. We are midway in our caregiving journey. This story has not reached the end, my caregiving will continue for as long as it takes. Even with all the difficulties and challenges I still love my wife and will continue to do my best for her.

True Love Cares.

True Calling
Laura Marie Patterson

Chapter 9 Dave – A Family Caregiver's Perspective

Related Resources

Appendix F: Working with Family Members   182

Appendix H: Caring for the Caregiver   194

Related Chapters

Chapter 2: Jimmy and Sabrina - Their Commitment   14

Appendix A
Building Trusting Relationships

True Calling
Laura Marie Patterson

One of the first challenges caregivers confront in the home is the need to build rapport with a client. Rapport involves establishing a level of trust and open communication such that a client feels comfortable discussing their central and intimate concerns. Although caregivers sometimes form an instant rapport, the therapeutic relationship is typically established over time, through a number of contacts. The evolution of this process may be thought of as a "courtship period" in which the caregiver and client gradually become familiar with each other and gain a sense of each others values and priorities. Ideally, the relationship between caregiver and client is transformed through this process so that the caregiver, who was formerly a guest in the client's home, becomes a trusted friend and adviser.

10 tips to enhance rapport and to build trust:

• Have good eye contact
• Demonstrate empathy, warmth, respect, and genuineness.
• Be consistent and persistent and follow through on promises
• Give the client a sense of control
• Acknowledge difficult feelings
• Share humor and laugh at jokes
• Share personal experiences
• Avoid questioning or challenging
• Lean forward - be attentive and show interest
• Use gestures and positive body language

The important thing to remember is that trust takes time and that it is earned and not given. Realize that there may have been mistrust that was fostered by a previous caregiver or family member. In those cases, rebuilding trust in a new caregiver will be even more challenging for the client. The best way to begin the rebuilding process is with open and honest communication concerning your clients fears and concerns. By becoming an active listener and supporting your clients emotions you become a key component to your clients recovery, earning their confidence and trust.

Examples of activities that foster good client/caregiver relationships:

Look through the clients family photo albums with them. Show interest by asking about the people in the pictures and the events depicted. If the photos are disorganized and not in albums, suggest helping them to build scrapbooks. This is a great shared activity and may help with the client's memory.

Sharing in activities that your client enjoys. Crossword puzzles, jigsaw puzzles, boardgames or just listening to music or watching T.V. Spending your time together in a fun and constructive way is the best way to build rapport and pass the time of day with a shared feeling of accomplishment.

When taking walks together, communicate. Even small talk can lead to positive and full-filling conversations. Walking and talking is good exercise and a great relationship building activity. Encourage the client to take the lead in the conversation by asking questions about the neighborhood or other visuals that you may encounter while on your walks.

True Calling
Laura Marie Patterson

Conversation Topics You Should Avoid:

Sharing your religious or political views with your client is strongly discouraged. These topics can cause friction because of possible opposing view-points. If your client asks your opinion on such topics, keep your answers short and neutral. Often times the client is asking these pointed questions in an effort to "size you up" and to form a moral opinion.

Keep your personal life private and never share your marital or financial problems with your client. You are there to support your clients physical and emotional needs and not the other way around. Always stay professional. Support and do not burden your client with your own issues.

Never share your personal address or phone number with your client unless it is required in the course of your duties. Having your spouse, friends or other family members visit you while at your clients home is not a good idea. Depending on the relationship that you have established over time, some social activities between your family and the client may be shared.

Laura Marie Patterson, Author

Appendix B
Safety in the Home and Hidden Dangers

True Calling
Laura Marie Patterson

One of the first things you should do when starting with a new client is make an assessment of possible hazards or safety issues within their home. Depending on your clients age, disability or mental condition, the concerns will vary. If your client is independent enough to be left home alone at night, it is your responsibility to insure that the home is safe and secure before leaving.

It is highly recommended that a lifeline or other medical alert device is available for your client and is within reach at all times during your absence. In addition, assess your clients mental and physical condition to be sure that they are capable of staying alone without supervision. Certain medications can cause confused states and you need to be fully aware of what medications your client is taking and that they are being taken according to the container's directions. A divided pill box is the best way to monitor your clients medications and that they are not a missing a dosage. The remaining medications should then be stored in a safe place away from your client's reach.

Another precaution would be to have emergency lighting within easy reach of your client in case of a power failure. Strategically placed flashlights or battery powered lanterns by the bedside and in each of the rooms are highly recommenced. Also make sure that the batteries are fresh and that they remain in working order.

It is important for you to establish a sense of security for your client that translates to confidence and trust in your abilities. One way you can accomplish this goal is to always communicate your concerns for their welfare and safety. Explain the reasons for any corrections that need to be made to their home as a suggestion for their own personal safety and your piece of mind as their caregiver. Involving your client in the discovery process of these safety concerns is a great way to build rapport and validate the necessity for making the changes.

Once you have identified any safety issues or hidden hazards in the clients home, the next step is to develop an emergency action plan in case of earthquake, fire or other unforeseen disaster. Knowing what to do in the case of emergency will save valuable minutes and can mean the difference between life and death. Go over this plan with your client if possible. Get the names of friends and neighbors that could be of service in an emergency and most importantly know your clients primary care physicians name and phone number. In a medical emergency always call 911 first before taking any other action.

Safety Checklist For Your Clients Home

_____Emergency numbers are posted by each telephone.

_____Medical Alert (Personal Emergency Response Systems) if Needed.

_____Inside and outside door handles and locks are easy to operate.

_____Windows open easily from the inside and they have a secure locking system

_____The water heater thermostat is not set above 120 degrees F to prevent scalding.

_____Medications are stored in a safe place, not expired and are clearly marked.

_____Carpeting and rugs are not worn or torn and that no trip risks are present.

_____Small, loose rugs have non-skid backing and are not placed in traffic areas.

_____Appliances, lamps and cords are clean and in good condition.

_____Electrical cords are out of the flow of traffic and not underneath rugs and furniture.

_____Smoke alarms are present and are in working order. Check batteries regularly.

_____The bathtub or shower has a non-skid mat or strips on the standing area.

_____Grab bars are installed on the walls by the bathtub and toilet.

_____A lamp or flashlight is kept within reach of your client's bed.

_____A night-light is used to brighten the way to the bathroom at night.

_____Plenty of room to walk around furniture and exits and doorways are clear.

Laura Marie Patterson, Author

Appendix C
Nutrition and Food Preparation

True Calling
Laura Marie Patterson

The task of meal planning and food preparation can feel overwhelming to caregivers. There are many cultural values and preferences around food. You may wish to ask yourself the following questions:

•What is a healthy diet? Unhealthy diet?
•What foods or food groups must be included in the daily diet?
•What foods are appropriate at different stages of the life span?
•What are my foods likes and dislikes? Why?
•What are my food taboos?
•What foods do I eat for celebrations?

Be aware that your client may answer those questions quite differently than you due to their own traditions and preferences. Respect for those preferences is of utmost importance.

Nutrition for the elderly is important as their health declines due to the aging process. Physiological changes occur slowly over time in all body systems. In addition, illnesses, life events, their genetic predisposition and socioeconomic factors need to be considered. Eating a balanced diet rich in whole grains, low in fats, with sufficient servings of fruits and vegetables offers a sound basis. Obviously, the clients overall health history needs to be taken into consideration when you are planning and preparing food for the client. Chronic diseases such as diabetes, hypertension, atherosclerosis (thickening of the artery due to build up of plaque), will dictate specific dietary requirements. Additionally, if your client has had a stroke, he or she may need structural changes in the food such as a mechanical soft diet.

Regardless of specific needs, best practices always include implementing as many *whole, natural foods* into the diet as possible. The science of nutrition is always in debate. New studies come out with recommendations and then those recommendations may change due to new research. There has never been any debate about the value of simple, whole foods, and any caregiver can cut an apple, slice fresh pineapple, steam some asparagus, or trim some fresh green beans! Buying fresh fruits and vegetables that are in season and introducing them one at a time can provide variety which often is lacking in the diets of seniors, who often eat the same foods over and over again. Due to the aging process, seniors can have a loss of smell and taste. If food doesn't smell or taste good, they may not be willing to try it. For example, overcooking vegetables until they are mushy aren't as appealing as a crunchy raw green bean for some.

Seniors have decreased calorie needs as they age. Many of them have a decrease in activity and less lean muscle mass. It's wise to purchase and serve lower calorie items that are high in nutrients because they need less calories and food volume. Also, vitamin and mineral needs continue to be important throughout the lifespan. Again, serving a variety of foods generally can meet the requirements. Eating five servings of fruits and vegetables per day is a good rule of thumb.

True Calling
Laura Marie Patterson

Involving the client in the planning process as much as possible is respectful and also promotes client "buy in" for healthy eating. Perhaps looking through the newspaper for specials and/or finding coupons for foods you normally buy is a suggestion. Making a shopping list and getting the client out to the supermarket gives the client a chance to participate in the process and has other benefits such as community engagement and exercise. It may be best to shop when the store is not crowded. If the client has a computer, you could also include them in online shopping. Any activity that promotes client engagement is of value. The U.S. Food and Drug Administration have a Modified Food Pyramid for older adults that can be used as an interactive tool for meal planning with the senior. If the senior cannot do it with the caregiver, it can be a useful tool for the caregiver. The food pyramid could be drawn onto a large piece of paper and specific foods could be drawn or cut out of magazines and glued down. The food pyramid has all the major food groups represented with 8 glasses of water for hydration reminders. At the base of the pyramid is a visual reminder of the need to exercise.

Try getting creative to make mealtime more pleasant. Some suggestions are eating by a window, eating lunch at a park, attending nutrition programs for the elderly at community center, inviting others over, and adding special touches to your dinner setting such as flowers, candles, etc.

Contributed by Kimberly Wilcox
RN, BSN, MA – Care Manager.

Appendix D
Dementia and Memory Loss

True Calling
Laura Marie Patterson

A loved one with dementia poses many challenges for families and caregivers. People with dementia from conditions such as Alzheimer's and related diseases have a progressive brain disorder that makes it more and more difficult for them to remember things, think clearly, communicate with others, or take care of themselves. In addition, dementia can cause mood swings and even change a person's personality and behavior. This resource provides some practical strategies for dealing with the troubling behavior problems and communication difficulties often encountered when caring for a person with dementia.

We are not born knowing how to communicate with a person with dementia, but we can learn. Improving your communication skills will help make caregiving less stressful and will likely improve the quality of your relationship with your loved one or client. Good communication skills will also enhance your ability to handle the difficult behavior you may encounter as you care for a person with a dementing illness.

Tip #1. Set a positive mood for interaction. Your attitude and body language communicate your feelings and thoughts stronger than your words. Set a positive mood by speaking to your loved one in a pleasant and respectful manner. Use facial expressions, tone of voice and physical touch to help convey your message and show your feelings of affection.

Tip #2 Get the person's attention. Limit distractions and noise turn off the radio or TV, close the curtains or shut the door, or move to quieter surroundings. Before speaking, make sure you have her attention; address her by name, identify yourself by name and relation, and use nonverbal cues and touch to help keep her focused. If she is seated, get down to her level and maintain eye contact.

Tip #3 State your message clearly. Use simple words and sentences. Speak slowly, distinctly and in a reassuring tone. Refrain from raising your voice higher or louder; instead, pitch your voice lower. If she doesn't understand the first time, use the same wording to repeat your message or question. If she still doesn't understand, wait a few minutes and rephrase the question. Use the names of people and places instead of pronouns or abbreviations.

Tip #4 Ask simple, answerable questions. Ask one question at a time; those with yes or no answers work best. Refrain from asking open-ended questions or giving too many choices. For example, ask, "Would you like to wear your white shirt or your blue shirt?" Better still, show her the choices—visual prompts and cues also help clarify your question and can guide her response.

Tip #5 Listen with your ears, eyes and heart. Be patient in waiting for your loved one's reply. If she is struggling for an answer, it's okay to suggest words. Watch for nonverbal cues and body language, and respond appropriately. Always strive to listen for the meaning and feelings that underlie the words.

True Calling
Laura Marie Patterson

Tip #6   Break down activities into a series of steps. This makes many tasks much more manageable. You can encourage your loved one to do what he can, gently remind him of steps he tends to forget, and assist with steps he's no longer able to accomplish on his own. Using visual cues, such as showing him with your hand where to place the dinner plate, can be very helpful.

Tip #7   When the going gets tough, distract and redirect. When your loved one becomes upset, try changing the subject or the environment. For example, ask him for help or suggest going for a walk. It is important to connect with the person on a feeling level, before you redirect. You might say, "I see you're feeling sad—I'm sorry you're upset. Let's go get something to eat."

Tip #8   Respond with affection and reassurance. People with dementia often feel confused, anxious and unsure of themselves. Further, they often get reality confused and may recall things that never really occurred. Avoid trying to convince them they are wrong. Stay focused on the feelings they are demonstrating (which are real) and respond with verbal and physical expressions of comfort, support and reassurance. Sometimes holding hands, touching, hugging and praise will get the person to respond when all else fails.

Tip #9   Remember the good old days. Remembering the past is often a soothing and affirming activity. Many people with dementia may not remember what happened 45 minutes ago, but they can clearly recall their lives 45 years earlier. Therefore, avoid asking questions that rely on short-term memory, such as asking the person what they had for lunch. Instead, try asking general questions about the person's distant past—this information is more likely to be retained.

Tip #10.   Maintain your sense of humor. Use humor whenever possible, though not at the person's expense. People with dementia tend to retain their social skills and are usually delighted to laugh along with you.

Handling Troubling Behavior

Some of the greatest challenges of caring for a loved one with dementia are the personality and behavior changes that often occur. You can best meet these challenges by using creativity, flexibility, patience and compassion. It also helps to not take things personally and maintain your sense of humor.

Caring for a loved one with dementia poses many challenges for families and caregivers. People with dementia from conditions such as Alzheimer's and related diseases have a progressive brain disorder that makes it more and more difficult for them to remember things, think clearly, communicate with others, or take care of themselves. In addition, dementia can cause mood swings and even change a person's personality and behavior. This Fact Sheet provides some practical strategies for dealing with the troubling behavior problems and communication difficulties often encountered when caring for a person with dementia.

What works today, may not tomorrow. The multiple factors that influence troubling behaviors and the natural progression of the disease process means that solutions that are effective today may need to be modified tomorrow—or may no longer work at all. The key to managing difficult behaviors is being creative and flexible in your strategies to address a given issue.

True Calling
Laura Marie Patterson

Get support from others. You are not alone—there are many others caring for someone with dementia. Call your local Area Agency on Aging, the local chapter of the Alzheimer's Association, a Caregiver Resource Center or one of the groups listed below in Resources to find support groups, organizations and services that can help you. Expect that, like the loved one you are caring for, you will have good days and bad days. Develop strategies for coping with the bad days.

Contributed by Beth Logan, M.S.W.
Education and Training Consultant and Specialist in Dementia Care.

Appendix E
Exercise and Social Activities

True Calling
Laura Marie Patterson

Try to engage in activities that your client is familiar with, such as, socializing, board games, scrap-booking, crafts, cooking, horseshoe, exercising and other fun events rather than teaching a new skill that would promote frustration.

The activities you select should encourage memory retention and increase self-worth. Therefore, seat down with your loved one for several minutes a day, and compile a list of what your client enjoys doing.

Make an effort to schedule these activities at the same time each day, so it is expected and looked forward to as a routine.

Here are some suggestions:

Socializing

Invite family members and friends to your visit client. Make sure your client consent to the guest visiting. You don't want to agitate or frustrate your client with someone who isn't pleasant. Brief your guest on certain subjects to bring up prior to arriving. Suggest positive topics and enjoyable moments from the past. Another social interaction activity would be to play with a pet, such as a dog or cat. Pet therapy has demonstrated a great benefit. Take your client to a pet park to meet with family members, neighbors, and other friends.

Games For Seniors

There are many board and card games that your your client may have played in the past. Ask for their top 5 favorite games, and rotate them each week during game time. Just make sure the game is not frustrating and complicated at this stage of dementia or Alzheimer's. Encourage games that stimulate the memory process and agility.

Scrap-booking for Seniors

Scrap-booking is another fun activity to entertain your loved one. It also can assist with memory retention and self-esteem. Gather old family pictures and organize them into family functions, such as birthdays, vacations, holidays and other family events. This will be a great time to spend with your loved one while going down memory lane. There may be local scrap-booking classes at craft stores or at your senior community center to assist you. Scrap-booking is a great way to journal many memories for your client and to have a great time with your.

Crafts

Making crafts is another great time to spend with client. Plan a week or two ahead of what you're going to make, such as a beaded necklace, colored bath salt jars, hand print craft, write a poem and make a craft frame for it or assemble a model car, boat or plane. Make sure you have all the supplies needed to complete the project. It would be very frustrating for your client if they can't complete their craft project.

Painting

Painting may help your client express themselves at this point of their lives. You can make the painting project large or small. For example, your client could assist with painting one of the rooms in the home, or paint a smaller project, such as, a portrait of the tree in your garden. Painting is very stimulating, and it may trigger fond memories for client. It will give them a since of accomplishment and boost their self-esteem.

True Calling
Laura Marie Patterson

Dancing

Dancing is another great activity that improves client's physical and mental well being. Studies show dancing improves mental capacity because it requires split second decision making. Discuss enrolling into a dance class with your client . Many community organizations host dancing classes, such as, senior community centers, community colleges or take private dancing classes at a local studio.

Exercising

Maintaining physical shape is also important for your client and yourself. Exercising may promote sleeping behavior, physical stamina, flexibility, balancing and decrease agitation and depression associated with Alzheimer's disease or dementia. Therefore, you should incorporate an exercise program into your client 's daily schedule.

The exercise program should consist of mixed activities that are fun and social for both of you, for example, do some gardening around the home, walking around the block, do swimming pool exercises, play badminton, table tennis, Tai Shi or other exercise programs. Some programs can be viewed on your local PBS Network, and others can be checked out from the library in the form of a DVD.

There are local organizations that may have an exercise program for seniors, such as, your local senior center, YMCA, and other private gyms. There are also certified personal trainers that specialize in senior exercises, and can come into your home to implement the program. Discuss the plan with your your client and primary physician prior to starting any exercise plan. You want to be sure your loved one can tolerate the physical activities.

Cooking

Cooking with your client could be a wonderful time to spend together. Always have them involved in the meal selection but limit the choices. Physicians and dietitians encourage healthy meals and snacks that are stimulating to the senses, for example, use multi-colored food choices with familiar taste and smell from the persons past.

You should allow enough time for meal preparation, eating time and socializing.

Many experts suggest to having quiet meals at the same time everyday. However, other healthcare professionals recommend soft background music of your loved one choice or nature music while eating. These environmental modifications may encourage positive eating behaviors and memory stimulation. It may also reduce agitation and aggression. Therefore, you may want to talk about this option with client. Also, constructive encouragement is also a must during meal time.

Music & Singing

Music is good for the soul. Therefore, develop a list of songs or music compositions that your client enjoy listening to, and download it to a CD, MP3 player or other multimedia devices for future listening. your client may love singing church hymns or other songs. Take a few moments during the week to sing familiar songs. They may have played an instrument in the past. Encourage them to play a sing along. Music is known to reduce anxiety, delusion and aggression. It also relaxes your client and assists with pain management. Therefore, try to schedule time for music and singing on a regular basis.

True Calling
Laura Marie Patterson

Reading & Story Telling

Set aside some time during the day for reading. Compile a list of books that your client enjoys reading. You can also take them to your local community library to help chose the best books. Additionally, you may ask them to tell a story from the book they read. This activity helps recall and communication skills. Many professionals say, "If you don't use it, you'll lose it." Therefore, encourage this activity on a consistent basis.

Laura Marie Patterson, Author

Appendix F
Working With Family Members

True Calling
Laura Marie Patterson

As a professional caregiver, you will often be confronted with issues concerning your client and their families. It is important to remember that all families have a dynamic and it is best to avoid becoming involved with family politics unless absolutely necessary. It is also important for an effective caregiver to communicate openly with the clients family.

It is understandable that the clients family would wish to be kept inform of any issues that would arise during the course of their loved ones care. Effective caregiving requires on going communication and interaction with the clients family and most importantly confidentiality with information that is shared. This includes privileged conversations between you and your client or with the clients family members.

Here are some simple tips for effectively communicating with the clients family.

• Be an active listener.
Family members know their loved one and can be very helpful with educating you with the likes, dislikes and mood points concerning your client. This also works in reverse, as clients sometimes have difficulty in communicating their needs to family members.

• Be a facilitator and not a wedge.
As a caregiver you have a responsibility to both your clients physical and emotional well being. It is for this reason that you listen to your clients family concerns and communicate them effectively. You are not a judge of who is right or wrong. You are a messenger so that the family is made aware of any client issues that may need attention.

•Don't take family issues personally

Try not to take it personally if family members are frustrated, angry, critical or if communication is difficult. Try to keep things in perspective and focus on the things you can change and not on those you cannot. Working closely with families in their own homes demands good communication, relationship, negotiation, goal-setting and conflict management skills.

•Take the appropriate action if family abuse is suspected.

This is a a very important duty for a caregiver as you spend time with your client and are aware of their psychological and physical changes. Elder abuse happens with the family more often than with outside influences. You are required by law to report any suspected abuse to the proper authorities. These reports are kept confidential.

The protocol for reporting observed abuse or if your client requires social intervention in family matters depends on if you are working independently or through an agency. If you are an employee of a caregiving agency, then follow the established procedure as set forth in your employee handbook or other guideline. As a independently contracted caregiver you will need to report these issues to your local social services. There are family support services that may arrange counseling for your client and their family if needed. The best rule is to observe, evaluate and report any suspected abuse.

True Calling
Laura Marie Patterson

Sharing in the care of your client with family members:

There are some cases where you may share in the responsibility of your clients care along with one or more of their family members. Communication with the caring family member is key. If your shift is to begin in the morning when the family member leaves for work, you must either communicate verbally or at very least by leaving notes for each other. A plain note book with the date and time of important events concerning the care of your client is a effective tool to communicate issues. Writing notes in a diary format is very helpful for both the family caregiver and yourself. Knowing the mood and or physical condition of your client the previous evening is essential in planning for the days care.

In any case, a good working relationship with your clients family either by telephone or in person is beneficial and necessarily. Open and honest discussions about your clients care with family members builds a trusting relationship and instils confidence in your ability to care for their loved one.

Laura Marie Patterson, Author

Appendix G
Supporting Loss and Grief

True Calling
Laura Marie Patterson

Grief is a natural process, an intense fundamental emotion, a universal experience which makes us human. It is a process that entails extremely hard work over a period of many painful months or years. People grieve because they are deprived of a loved one; the sense of loss is profound. The loss of a spouse, child, or parent affects our very identities—the way we define ourselves as a husband, wife, parent, or offspring. Moreover, grief can arise from the survivor's sudden change in circumstances after a death and the fear of not knowing what lies ahead.

The death of someone close can be a life-changing experience. If you are the primary caregiver of someone you love, this experience can affect every aspect of your life for some time. It is natural to grieve the death of a loved one before, during, and after the actual time of their passing. The process of accepting the unacceptable is what grieving is all about.

•Anticipatory Grief

If someone has had a prolonged illness or serious memory impairment, family members may begin grieving the loss of the person's "former self" long before the time of death. This is sometimes referred to as "anticipatory grief." Anticipating the loss, knowing what is coming, can be just as painful as losing a life. Family members may experience guilt or shame for "wishing it were over" or seeing their loved one as already "gone" intellectually. It is important to recognize these feelings as normal. Ultimately, anticipatory grief is a way of allowing us to prepare emotionally for the inevitable.

Preparing for the death of a loved one can allow family members to contemplate and clear unresolved issues and seek out the support of spiritual advisers, family, and friends. And, depending on the impaired person's intellectual capacity, this can be a time to identify your loved one's wishes for burial and funeral arrangements.

•Sudden Loss

A death that happens suddenly and unexpectedly is an immeasurable tragedy. This type of loss often generates shock and confusion for loved ones left behind. Incidents such as a fatal accident, heart attack, or suicide can leave family members perplexed and searching for answers. In these cases, family members may be left with unresolved issues, such as feelings of guilt that can haunt and overwhelm a grieving person. These feelings may seem to take over your life at first. But over time it is possible to get past these thoughts and forgive yourself and your loved one. Give yourself plenty of time; it's virtually impossible to make yourself "move on" before you're ready.

How Long Does Grieving Last?

Grief impacts each individual differently. Recent research has shown that intense grieving lasts from three months to a year and many people continue experiencing profound grief for two years or more. Others' response to this extended grieving process may sometimes cause people to feel there is something wrong with them or they are behaving abnormally. This is not the case. The grieving process depends on the individual's belief system, religion, life experiences, and the type of loss suffered.

True Calling
Laura Marie Patterson

Prolonged bereavement is not unusual. Many people find solace in seeking out other grievers or trusted friends. However, if feelings of being overwhelmed continue over time, professional support should be sought.

•Symptoms of Grief

Grief can provoke both physical and emotional symptoms, as well as spiritual insights and turmoil.

Physical symptoms include low energy or exhaustion, headaches, or upset stomach. Some people will sleep excessively; others may find they are pushing themselves to extremes at work. These activity changes may make an individual more prone to illness. It is important to take care of yourself during this period of bereavement by maintaining a proper diet, exercise, and rest. Taking care of your body can help heal the rest of you, even if you do not feel inclined to do so.

Emotional symptoms include memory gaps, distraction or preoccupation, irritability, depression, euphoria, wailing rages, and passive resignation. Some people identify strongly with the person who died and his/her feelings. If you have experienced a loss and are hurting it is reasonable that your responses may seem "unreasonable." Nonetheless, it is important not to judge yourself too harshly as you experience conflicting and overwhelming emotions.

Like grief itself, people's coping strategies vary. Some people cope best through quiet reflection, others seek exercise or other distractions. Some have a tendency to engage in reckless or self-destructive activities (e.g., excessive drinking). It is vital to obtain support in order to regain some sense of control and to work through your feelings.

A trained counselor, support group, or trusted friend can help you sort through feelings such as anxiety, loss, anger, guilt, and sadness. If depression or anxiety persists, a doctor or psychiatrist may prescribe antidepressant drugs to help alleviate feelings of hopelessness.

Spiritual experiences include grieving which may make you feel closer to God and allow you to be more open to religious experiences than ever before. Conversely, many people express anger or outrage at God. You may feel cut off from God or from your own soul altogether—a temporary paralysis of the spirit. If you are a person of faith, you may question your faith in God, in yourself, in others or in life. A member of the clergy or spiritual adviser can help you examine the feelings you are experiencing. Learning to deal with grief is learning to live again.

Stages of Grief

Often portrayed as a grief "wheel," these stages do not necessarily follow a set order.

- Shock
- Emotional release
- Depression, loneliness, and a sense of isolation
- Physical symptoms of distress
- Feelings of panic
- A sense of guilt
- Anger or rage
- Inability to return to usual activities
- The gradual regaining of hope
- Acceptance as we adjust our lives to reality

True Calling
Laura Marie Patterson

Most people who have lost someone close go through all or some of these stages, although not necessarily in this specific order. This kind of healthy grieving can help a person move through a significant loss with minimal harm to self, either physical or mental.

When a person is confused, or otherwise unable to express preferences, family members are often put in the position of becoming surrogate decision makers. Such decisions present a thorny array of medical, legal, and moral questions. Decisions to provide or withhold life support are based on personal values, beliefs, and consideration for what the person might have wanted. Such decisions are painful. Family members should give themselves ample time to cope with these life and death decisions and to process feelings of doubt or blame which may surface.

Tips for Helping the Bereaved:

• Be available. Offer support in an unobtrusive but persistent manner.
• Listen without giving advice.
• Do not offer stories of your own. This can have the effect of dismissing the grieving person's pain.
• Allow the grieving person to express anger or bitterness, including such expressions against God. This may be normal behavior in an attempt to find meaning in what has happened.
• Realize that no one can undo the loss. To heal, the individual must endure the grief process. Allow him/her to feel the pain.
• Be patient, kind, and understanding without being patronizing. Don't claim to "know" what the other person is feeling.
• Don't force the individual to share feelings if he/she doesn't want to.

•Don't hesitate to share a hug or handclasp when appropriate. Physical and emotional touch can bring great comfort to the bereaved.

•Be there in the long run, when friends and family have all gone back to their routines.

•Remember holidays, birthdays, and anniversaries which have important meaning for the bereaved. Offer support during this time. Don't be afraid of reminding the person of the loss; he/she is already thinking about it.

Credits:

Managing Grief and Bereavement: A Guide for Families and Professionals Caring for Memory Impaired Adults and Other Chronically Ill Persons (booklet), 1993, Duke Family Support Program, Duke University Medical Center, Durham, NC 27710.

This page was left blank intentionally.

Appendix H
Caring for the Caregiver

True Calling
Laura Marie Patterson

Caregiving can be a wonderful and rewarding experience. It can also be extremely demanding both mentally and physically. The person you're caring for might well be your first priority, but all humans have limits. Helping yourself stand up to the demands you face is critical. You need to feel a sense of balance to maintain your well-being. So what can you do?

Let's start by looking at some simple things you can incorporate into your life that can go a long way toward your well-being. Remember, the goal is to relieve stress, not add to it. So use what works for you and the moment.

Take advantage of quick, simple pleasures – Step outside, soak in the sunshine, and breathe in the crisp, fresh air. Have a cup of calming herbal tea, inhaling the wonderful aroma. Put bouquets of flowers you love in all the main rooms. Listen to soothing, uplifting music. The list is endless.

Stay connected with others – Caregivers can get so absorbed in what they are doing that they can tend to isolate, often without knowing it. Feeling connected can be one of the most important things you can do to not feel alone. Spending time with others can be a strong stress reliever and great for your well-being.

"Buddy" with another caregiver – This is something many caregivers don't think about but can have a great impact. Who better than someone walking in your shoes to be able to understand what you're going through?

Care for your nutritional needs – The body needs good nutrition to function well. Planning a week's worth of balanced meals can make it much easier to eat well. There are many ways to eat well and not spend your day in the kitchen. You just need to experiment to see what works best for you.

Exercise – This is a natural stress reliever and a healthy way to live. Many caregivers give up exercise due to time. You might not have time to go to a health club, but don't let that stop you. You could watch a fitness DVD, do stretching exercises, tai chi, yoga, etc. Doing three ten-minute increments might work better for you than 30-minutes at one time.

Get enough rest – Your body needs adequate rest. Sleep isn't a luxury. You simply can't function without it. Make sure you get the rest you need.

Meditate – This is a great way to focus on your breathing, helping you to relax, as well as turning inward from the outside world. Regular meditation can have a cumulative effect on your outlook and peacefulness.

Read uplifting material – Inspiring poems, quotes, articles, and books can make you feel good and keep you positive.

Humor – You know the saying, "Laughter is the best medicine." Humor is a great stress reliever. Get as much as you can.

Journal your feelings – caregiving can be enormously demanding, involving a lot of mixed emotions. Expressing your feelings is wonderful for getting things "out of your system." Journaling is a great way to release stress and get you in touch with your deepest feelings.

Focus on gratitude – Listing what you enjoy about being a caregiver, as well as what you are grateful for in your life, can be a very gratifying, uplifting, and meaningful tool. It's nice to read to keep your spirits high during difficult days.

True Calling
Laura Marie Patterson

Support groups – There is no need to go it alone. A caregiver support group can provide you with lots of support, an avenue to express your feelings with those who understand, and a chance to hear the experiences of others.

Use respite care – We all need to take time for ourselves and rejuvenate. Make a list of people who might enable you to take a break outside the home. Think of your family, friends, neighbors, community members, and others. People are often more than happy to help if asked. Professionals are always available as well and can be a great resource.

By thinking creatively and listing ways you can incorporate more balance into your life will make it more likely to happen. Many people feel selfish or guilty by making themselves a priority while being a caregiver. Don't fall into that trap. You're human and have your needs also. Do you really want someone physically exhausted and mentally drained caring for your loved one?

Contributed by Pam Alberts, MSW, LICSW, CEP, MBA

Internet Resources

Caregiver Resources

www.caregiving.org

• Offers Free Online Caregiving Courses.
• Nationwide Database of Care Resources.
• Bookstore with Caregiving Publications.

National Family Caregiver's Association

www.nfacares.org

The National Family Caregivers Association educates, supports, and empowers more than 65 million Americans who care for loved ones with a chronic illness, disability or the frailties of old age.

Caregiver Resource Network

www.caregiverresource.net

Providing information and support for family and professional caregivers. There is also a number of free pod casts available.

AGIS – Eldercare, Long Term Care and Caregiving Resources

www.agis.com

Helps caregivers and their loved ones meet the challenges of aging. Search local resources for facilities, care providers and government resources. Informative articles on caregiving and health related issues.

Acknowledgments

A heartfelt thanks to all that have made this book possible. Special thanks to my family and friends, whose encouragement and love kept my focus in the mist of so many distractions.

To my professional colleagues, some of which have become close friends during the course of this project. Your knowledge and insight within the resource chapters were invaluable contributions.

Kimberly Wilcox, RN, BSN, MA
Care Manager.

Beth Logan, M.S.W.
Education and Training Consultant and Specialist in Dementia Care.

Pam Alberts, MSW, LICSW, CEP, MBA

Managing Grief and Bereavement: A Guide for Families and Professionals Caring for Memory Impaired Adults and Other Chronically Ill Persons (booklet), 1993, Duke Family Support Program, Duke University Medical Center, Durham, NC 27710.

Finally, but never forgotten, the many special clients that I was given the gift of sharing in their lives. Your inspirational spirits will live forever within the pages of this book.

Laura Marie Patterson

This page was left blank intentionally.

www.ingramcontent.com/pod-product-compliance
Lightning Source LLC
Chambersburg PA
CBHW060849280326
41934CB00007B/977